Making a difference 2

The authors

Elisa Aguirre is a research assistant at North East London Foundation Trust (NELFT), which runs the maintenance CST trial as part of the SHIELD programme. Elisa is developing her PhD at University College London (UCL) based on the development and evaluation of the programme.

Dr Aimée Spector was the lead researcher in the original developed CST trial, since then she has published extensive research papers in relation to old age psychology, the CST training manual and leads the CST training course. She is now a Senior Lecturer in Clinical Psychology at University College London (UCL).

Amy Streater is a research assistant at North East London Foundation Trust (NELFT), which runs the maintenance CST trial. Amy is developing her PhD at University College London (UCL) based on the implementation into practice of the programme.

Dr Juanita Hoe is currently employed as a Senior Clinical Research Associate at University College London (UCL) coordinating the SHIELD programme. She is a psychiatric nurse by background and has substantial clinical and research experience involving people with dementia.

Professor Bob Woods is Professor of Clinical Psychology of Older People at the University of Wales Bangor and co-director of the Dementia Services Development Centre Wales. He has published extensive academic papers in relation to old age psychology and is editor of the journal Aging and Mental Health.

Professor Martin Orrell is Professor of Ageing and Mental Health at University College London (UCL) and a Consultant Old Age Psychiatrist at North East London Foundation Trust. He leads the SHIELD research programme on psychosocial interventions for dementia care. He has published over 150 academic papers and is editor of the journal Aging and Mental Health.

Making a difference 2

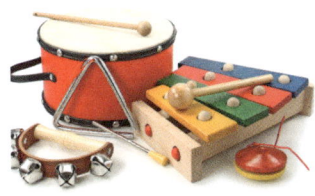
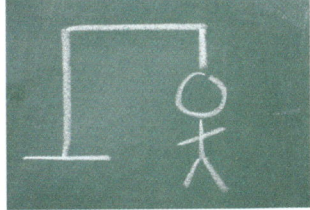
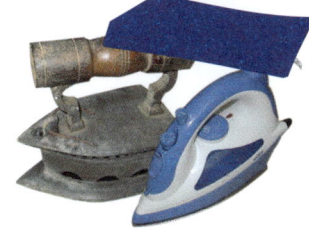
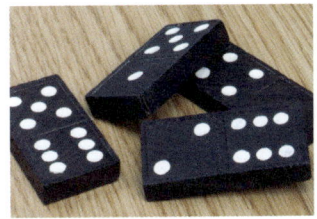
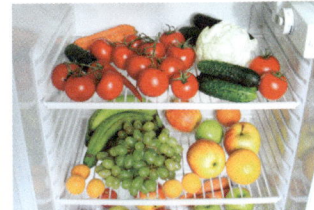
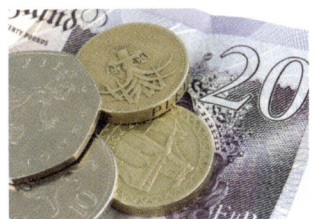
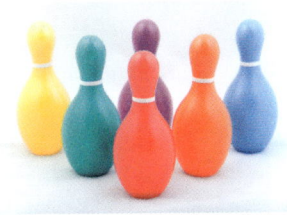
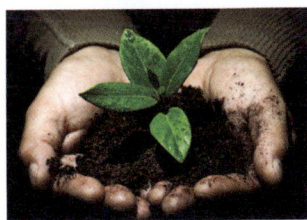
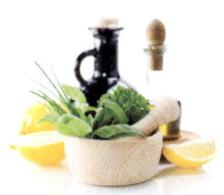

An evidence-based group programme
to offer maintenance cognitive stimulation therapy
(CST) to people with dementia

The manual for group leaders

VOLUME TWO

Elisa Aguirre, Aimée Spector, Amy Streater
Juanita Hoe, Bob Woods, Martin Orrell

Published by **The Journal of Dementia Care**

Making a difference 2

An evidence-based group programme to offer maintenance cognitive stimulation therapy (CST) to people with dementia
The manual for group leaders
Volume Two

First published in 2012
Reprinted 2012

Hawker Publications Culvert House, Culvert Road, London SW11 5DH

Tel: 020 7720 2108
Fax: 020 7498 3023
Website: www.careinfo.org

© 2012 UCL Unit of Mental Health Sciences, University College London and Dementia Services Development Centre Wales, University of Bangor

Copy editor: Kate Hawkins
Printed and bound in Great Britain by Information Press, Oxford

The right of Elisa Aguirre, Aimée Spector, Amy Streater, Juanita Hoe, Bob Woods and Martin Orrell to be identified as the authors of this work has been asserted by them in accordance with the Copyright, Designs and Patents Act 1988.

All rights reserved. This publication contains pages that may be photocopied. However, unless specified on the page, no part of this publication may be reproduced transmitted in any form or by any means, electronic or mechanical, including photocopy, recording, or any information storage and retrieval system without permission in writing from the publishers.

British Library Cataloguing in Publication Data
A catalogue record for this book is available from the
British Library
ISBN 978 1 874790 99 0

Book design by Prepare to Publish Ltd
mail@preparetopublish.com

Also published by Hawker Publications:
Making a Difference
Aimee Spector, Lene Thorgrimsen, Bob Woods, Martin Orrell
2006 ISBN 978 1 874790 78 5
For contact details see above

MAKING A DIFFERENCE 2 | # Contents

CST key principles Dr Aimée Spector — **7**

Maintenance CST programme — **12**
- Maintenance CST — 12
- How to use this manual — 13
- Managing and structuring maintenance sessions — 14
- Maintenance CST materials and equipment — 14
- Monitoring progress — 14
- Guidance for co-facilitators — 16

Maintenance CST sessions — **17**
- Session 1: My life (life history) — 18
- Session 2: Current affairs — 20
- Session 3: Food — 22
- Session 4: Being creative — 24
- Session 5: Number games — 26
- Session 6: Team games/quiz — 28
- Session 7: Sound — 30
- Session 8: Physical games — 32
- Session 9: Categorising objects — 34
- Session 10: Household treasures — 36
- Session 11: Useful tips (household tips) — 38
- Session 12: Thinking cards — 40
- Session 13: Visual clips discussion — 42
- Session 14: Art discussion — 44
- Session 15: Faces/scenes — 46
- Session 16: Word game — 48
- Session 17: Food (slogans/ads) — 50
- Session 18: Associated words — 52
- Session 19: Orientation — 54
- Session 20: Using money (video clips) — 56
- Session 21: Word game — 58
- Session 22: Household treasures — 59
- Session 23: My life (occupations) — 60
- Session 24: Useful tips — 62

References and further reading — **64**

Acknowledgements

Maintenance Cognitive Stimulation Programme (ISRCTN26286067) is part of the Support at Home - Interventions to Enhance Life in Dementia (SHIELD) project (Application No RP-PG-0606-1083) which is funded by the NIHR Programme Grants for Applied Research funding scheme. The grantholders are Professors Orrell (UCL), Woods (Bangor), Challis (Manchester), Moniz-Cook (Hull), Russell (Swansea), Knapp (LSE) and Dr Charlesworth (UCL).

This manual presents independent research commissioned by the National Institute for Health Research (NIHR) under its Programme Grants for Applied Research scheme (RP-PG-060-1083). The views expressed in this publication are those of the authors and not necessarily those of the NHS, the NIHR or the Department of Health.

We would like to thank the people with dementia, family caregivers, staff and professionals who took part in the development of the Maintenance Cognitive Stimulation programme through their participation in the focus groups and consensus conference.

The authors would also like to thank all of their SHIELD programme colleagues for their support and enthusiasm.

MAKING A DIFFERENCE 2 | CST key principles

This manual describes a specific programme of group activity and stimulation suitable for use with many people with dementia. You may have used, or be using many of these activities in your everyday work. What follows is an explanation of the key principles of cognitive stimulation therapy (CST), highlighting some of the ways in which CST may differ to other activities you do. It is important that all CST facilitators understand and put into practice the following principles. This section is essential!

> **Key Principles**
> 1 Mental stimulation
> 2 New ideas, thoughts and associations
> 3 Using orientation, sensitively and implicitly
> 4 Opinions, rather than facts
> 5 Using reminiscence, and as an aid to the here-and-now
> 6 Providing triggers to aid recall
> 7 Continuity and consistency between sessions
> 8 Implicit (rather than explicit) learning
> 9 Stimulating language
> 10 Stimulating executive functioning
> 11 Person-centred
> 12 Respect
> 13 Involvement
> 14 Inclusion
> 15 Choice
> 16 Fun
> 17 Maximising potential
> 18 Building / strengthening relationships

1. Mental stimulation

The first aim of CST is to mentally stimulate, in other words to get people's minds active and engaged. As everyone has different skills, some sessions will be more challenging for some people than for others. If people ask why things are difficult or seem concerned or anxious, it can be helpful to explain and reassure participants of this. You might explain that you are trying to get them to exercise skills that have not been used for a while, and stimulate different parts of the brain. It might help to explain that we now have evidence that this can improve cognitive functioning, making reference to the research. When you plan sessions, the aim is to pitch activities so that people have to make an effort, but that they are not too difficult, potentially making the person feel deskilled.

2. New ideas, thoughts and associations

Often we tend to talk about things from the past with people with dementia. Whilst this is enjoyable for people, it often involves recalling information which has been over-rehearsed. The aim of CST is to continually encourage new ideas, thoughts and associations, rather than just recall previously learned information. A good example of how to do this is in the 'faces' session. In typical group work, people might be shown a picture of a famous face and asked questions such as 'who is this'? 'what do you remember about them?'
In CST, participants are shown two or more pictures at once. The aim is to develop new ideas, thoughts and associations, through asking questions such as:
• What do these people have in common?
• How are they different?
• Who is the odd one out?
• Who would you rather be?
• Who is more attractive?
Similarly in the current affairs sessions, rather than introducing topics likely to have been discussed before (e.g. "What do you think of the royal family?"), people are encouraged to discuss new topics such as "Is modern art really art?" "What do you think of same sex weddings?".

3. Using orientation, sensitively and implicitly

Orientation is an important goal of CST, but the way that people are orientated is key. Rehearsal of orientation information (such as the date) and putting people on the spot with direct questions (e.g. "what is the address?") has in the past been described as demoralising. Orientation needs to be done in a subtle, implicit way at the beginning of each session. Orientation information such as the date, name of group and group members, activity of the day and news headline should always be written on a display board, and you might refer to the board in your discussion. When introducing the session and discussing something going on in the news, this is the time to subtly orientate people. For example, you might say "Do you think this weather is normal for October, or is it hotter / colder than usual?" "Is anyone's birthday around now?" Many of the activities provide scope for time orientation, for example you might make a collage with autumn leaves in 'Being creative' or bring in Christmas food in the 'Food' session.

4. Opinions rather than facts

In group sessions, we need to focus on people's strengths. If we focus on 'facts' too much, there is the risk that people will often be wrong. If we ask people for their opinions, then they may be amusing, sad, unusual, controversial or puzzling, but they cannot be wrong. Everyone in the group is entitled to their own opinion, of course. So, rather than say "Where did you go on holiday when you were a child?" (a memory question), ask "What's your favourite place to go on holiday?" or "Where would you advise a young family to go on holiday?" Rather than ask "Who is the Prime Minister", ask "What do you think of politicians?" or "Who has been the best leader of the country?" in the latter case giving a range of names, backed up by photographs. The group should never feel like a memory test. Avoid questions beginning "Who can remember…?".

5. Using reminiscence, and as an aid to the here and now

Using past memories is an excellent way of tapping into a strength that many people with dementia have, in terms of recalling experiences from much earlier in their lives. For many, it is also an enjoyable activity. Remember though that some people with dementia may have unhappy (even traumatic) memories of their earlier life, and some sensitivity is needed not to push members into exposing painful memories in the group setting. If a raw nerve is touched upon accidentally, take time with the person (on a one-to-one basis) to enable them to talk further, if they wish, or to regain their composure. The better that you know the backgrounds and life stories of group members, the less likely this is to occur, but unforeseeable areas of difficulty may still emerge. Reminiscence can also be a useful tool towards orientation, which is a key goal of CST. Many sessions allow you to compare old and new, thinking about how things have changed over time. For example, in 'Using money', you might discuss what you can buy for £10 now and what you could buy for £10 fifty years ago.

HINTS AND TIPS WHEN RUNNING CST GROUPS

6. Providing triggers and prompts to aid recall and concentration

The RO board is a useful way of triggering memories and aiding recall. Multi-sensory cues are also really important, as memory works much better if you do not rely on just one sense. There will be differences between members in their preferred sense – try to ensure a variety, so that there is a mix of activities involving vision, touch, hearing, taste and smell. Often it is a combination of senses that is most effective. For example, identifying sounds in the 'sounds' session is helped by looking at accompanying pictures, and the food session is enhanced if people can taste, smell and feel food with interesting textures (such as pineapples). Use non-verbal communication as well as verbal. Your facial expression, tone of voice, posture and gesture will speak volumes! For each individual having something to look at or touch really helps aid concentration. Words in a discussion may soon be lost when memory is limited; having the object, a photograph or picture keeps members' attention on the activity and encourages a group focus. Make multiple copies of materials, e.g. pictures in 'faces' and newspaper articles in 'current affairs', rather than passing one copy around.

7. Continuity and consistency between sessions

Memory and learning is supported through providing continuity and consistency between sessions. Examples of this include referring to the group name, always running groups in the same room and always starting sessions and ending sessions in a similar way (e.g. using warm-ups and songs).

8. Implicit (rather than explicit) learning

Ideally, people will not be too aware that they are learning and being stimulated, perceiving the groups more as 'fun activity groups'. A good example is the 'faces' session. People are not asked direct questions about names and facts related to individuals, but through more indirect questions relating to preferences and commonalities. As this happens, factual information tends to emerge without people feeling being 'put on the spot'.

9. Stimulating language

There is evidence from the research that language skills improve after CST. Many of the sessions stimulate language, for example naming of people and objects (e.g. in categorisation), thinking about word construction and word association.

10. Stimulating executive functioning

Executive functioning skills, particularly involving planning and organising, are often very impaired in dementia. There are several sessions which exercise these skills, for example planning and executing stages of a task (such as making a cake) in 'being creative'. Mental organisation is exercised through the discussion of similarities and differences in several sessions, word association and categorising objects.

11. Person centred

We need to see the person first and foremost, rather than focusing on the dementia and the associated impairments. Each person is unique, with a lifetime of experiences that have shaped their personality and attitudes, leading to a variety of skills, interests, preferences and abilities. Ask yourself about the person's strengths, rather than concentrating on their areas of difficulty. What will be appropriate and enjoyable for one person may be disliked intensely by another.

12. Respect

We need to show respect for the person, and never make them feel small or do anything to expose their difficulties in the group. Help the person to retain their dignity. People with dementia come from all types of cultural and religious backgrounds; show respect by getting to know what is important to each individual, and value the diversity of views, opinions and beliefs within a group. Allow people to be different.

13. Involvement

If during the group, you find yourself doing most of the talking, or talking 'at' the group, stop! Think about how you can get everyone involved, and offer choices of activities that will interest and engage your particular group. Encourage group members to address their contributions to each other, rather than everything being channelled through the group leader. Remember the group belongs to its members, not to the staff!

14. Inclusion

Watch out for individuals who appear isolated within the group. If this is due to hearing or vision problems, make arrangements for a leader to sit next to them to ensure they can join in, and make sure the person has their glasses or hearing aid, as appropriate. If the person is a little shy, encourage a more socially active group member to engage with them. If one person in the group has different views or opinions from all the other members, ensure they are not rejected or put down. Encourage an atmosphere where everyone's contribution is valued and respected, and diversity of views is welcomed.

15. Choice

This group programme is not prescriptive. It is fairly detailed simply to make life easier for group leaders, who will often have many other things on their minds apart from the group. Group members should always be offered choices, and alternative activities and approaches found if those offered here do not suit the needs and abilities of your particular group. Offering choices allows group members to become involved in making the group their own – selecting a name for the group, choosing music to use and so on. It goes without saying that no-one should be forced to participate in any particular activity. Those who are a little reluctant are most likely to be influenced by seeing others enjoying themselves rather than by being coerced. For each session, we have suggested a choice of activities, often geared to groups at different levels of ability or different interests. The activities have been organised according to how demanding they are on the person's memory and other cognitive skills. We've started with the first ones on the list as being the least demanding and the last ones on the list as being the more demanding. Choose which seems most appropriate for your group, or mix activities from the list or add your own ideas! There is space in the manual to note activities you have tried for each session, so that next time around they can be among the choices open to you.

16. Fun

Sometimes group members will comment 'this is like being back in school'. If they mean by this that they are being made to work hard in a strict and serious atmosphere, something is going wrong! The groups should provide a learning atmosphere which is fun and enjoyable, with a group of friends. Yes, members' brains should be stimulated, but so should their sense of humour! If members make comments about 'school', ask them what they liked and disliked about school, and reflect on whether the group leaders are taking on the role of 'teacher' too readily. Avoid using equipment that is, or looks like it is, intended for children (apart from when reminiscing about childhood). Group members are adults and we must ensure that nothing we do treats them like children.

17. Maximising potential

Be careful not to assume a person with dementia is unable to contribute or carry out an activity simply because they were not able to yesterday or last week. People with dementia often function at less than their full potential, perhaps due to lack of stimulation or opportunity. There is evidence that people with dementia can learn, with the right encouragement. This involves giving the person time, being careful not to overload or overwhelm them with information, and providing just enough prompting to enable the person to carry out the activity themselves. This will increase exposure to success, which also will aid learning and enjoyment. People with dementia are more likely to achieve their potential by doing rather than sitting passively and watching.

18. Building / strengthening relationships

The group sessions will help members get to know each other better, and can strengthen relationships between the members and leaders – especially if the leaders ensure they do not become 'teacher', but assist members, join in, have fun and don't present themselves as all-knowing experts. Person-centred care means allowing yourself to be a person, an ordinary human being, in person-to-person relationships with people with dementia. This is not necessarily easy, but in a small group, away from some of the care-giving pressures, it's possible and very worthwhile.

Dr Aimée Spector
Senior lecturer in clinical psychology
University College London (UCL)

MAKING A DIFFERENCE 2 | Maintenance CST programme

Maintenance Cognitive Stimulation Therapy (CST)

Cognitive Stimulation Therapy or 'CST' is a brief treatment for people with mild to moderate dementia. CST was designed following extensive evaluation of research evidence, hence it is an evidence-based treatment (Spector *et al*, 2003). The NICE guidance (NICE, 2006) on the management of dementia recommended the use of group cognitive stimulation for people with mild to moderate dementia, irrespective of drug treatments received. The basis of cognitive stimulation reflects the general view that lack of cognitive activity hastens cognitive decline, in normal ageing as well as in dementia (Breuil 1994; Small 2002). It also attempts to make use of the positive aspects of reality orientation, whilst ensuring that it is implemented in a properly sensitive and respectful manner (Spector 2001; Woods 2002). Clare *et al* (2004) have proposed the following definition for cognitive stimulation: engagement in a range of activities and discussions (usually in a group) aimed at general enhancement of cognitive and social functioning. CST targets cognitive and social functioning including current information and orientation in every session. The activities which are on offer in every session aim at generalised cognitive ability, rather than training in a specific cognitive modality, and are typically conducted in a group to enhance social functioning. CST treatment involves 14 sessions of themed activities, which run over a seven week period (see Making a Difference Manual; Spector *et al*, 2006).

We have found that continuing with weekly CST sessions helps to maintain the improvements in memory that were observed following the initial CST 14 session programme (Orrell *et al*, 2005). These maintenance sessions follow similar themes, but aim to use different materials wherever possible as it is important that boredom is avoided for both members and leaders. Each session's structure is the same as that for the initial CST sessions. The maintenance sessions have been developed using a review of the research evidence on cognitive stimulation and include additional themes not in the original CST programme (Aguirre *et al*, 2011).

A consensus conference was held in order to consult with professionals about a maintenance CST manual draft version 1. Focus groups were then undertaken to consult further about the second draft of the manual draft. These involved key stakeholders in the project. Separate groups were held for people with dementia, family carers and staff carers involved in running activities for people with dementia. The results from the focus groups led to further revision and the development of the final maintenance CST manual (Aguirre et al., 2011).

Maintenance CST sessions run once weekly over a 24-week period. Sessions aim to actively stimulate and engage people with dementia, whilst providing an optimal learning environment within the social benefits of a group. Just like CST sessions, maintenance CST can be administered by anyone working with people with dementia including care workers, occupational therapists and nurses. It is useful for the staff leading the sessions to have some experience running groups for people with dementia. Maintenance CST groups can take place in settings including residential homes, hospitals and/or day centres. They are planned to follow on from the completion of the 14 session seven week CST programme. To use this manual effectively you will need a copy of the original "Making a difference" manual which contains additional information about setting up and running groups.

How to use this manual

This manual provides a detailed guide to 24 sessions of Maintenance CST specifically designed to follow on after the completion of the (14 sessions) CST programme described in the Making a Difference manual (Spector *et al*, 2006). This manual describes each maintenance session and includes examples to get you started as a CST facilitator. The aim of this manual is for you to carry out one session per week for 24 weeks.

Each session is described on a separate page, so the session-by-session guide can be easily followed. The structure for each session follows that of the initial CST programme, which includes an opening activity, a main activity and the closing of each session. The activities for each session have been designed to stimulate each participant in the group and can be selected from a range of suggested tasks listed.

CST and maintenance CST themes development

CST Programme	Main theme	Maintenance CST programme
Session 1	Physical games	Session 8
Session 2	Sound	Session 7
Session 3	My life	Session 1 & 23
Session 4	Food	Session 3 & 17
Session 5	Current affairs	Session 2
Session 6	Faces/ scenes	Session 15
Session 7	Associated words, discussion	Session 18
Session 8	Being creative	Session 4
Session 9	Categorising objects	Session 9
Session 10	Orientation	Session 19
Session 11	Using money	Session 20
Session 12	Number game	Session 5
Session 13	Word game	Session 16 & 21
Session 14	Team games, quiz	Session 6
New maintenance	Useful tips	Session 11 & 24
New maintenance	Thinking cards	Session 12
New maintenance	Art discussion	Session 14
New maintenance	Visual Clips	Session 13
New maintenance	Household treasures	Session 10 & 22

Managing and structuring maintenance sessions

In all sessions make sure you have got the following:
- White board with orientation information (e.g. date, time, place)
- An introduction to the session where participants are warmly welcomed and helped to tune in to what is happening, including a brief reminder of what happened last session
- Warm up exercises related to the theme
- Main activity
- A closing where:
  – The work of the session is summed up
  – Suggestions are made for work at home
  – Personal and appreciative goodbyes.

Maintenance CST materials and equipment

A number of useful resources, including some of those used in this programme, are available from:

Speechmark Publishers Ltd
www.speechmark.net
Telford Road, Bicester, Oxfordshire OX26 4LQ
Tel: 01869 244644

Winslow
www.winslow-cat.com
Freepost NEA 11153, Chesterfield S40 2ZY
Tel: 01246 210416

The Robert Opie Collection – reminiscence
www.robertopiecollection.com

CST dementia website
www.cstdementia.com

SJB Associates
www.sjbassociates.org.uk/links/35-admin
12 Troon Avenue, Darlington, County Durham DL1 3HY

Making a difference manual
www.careinfo.org/books
Spector A, Thorgrimsen L, Woods B and Orrell M (2006). *Making a difference: An evidence-based group programme to offer Cognitive Stimulation therapy (CST) to people with dementia.* Hawker Publications, Culvert House, Culvert Road, London, SW11 5DH, UK.

Materials / Equipment

A list of items that you may want to purchase before starting CST groups (* indicates these are essential – others are open to improvisation):

- Whiteboard and pens *
- Soft ball *
- CD player *
- Song books *
- CDs of music enjoyed by group members *
- Skittles / indoor bowls / boules
- Sound effects CDs
- Old fashioned toys (e.g. spinning top, jacks, hoopla) - may be borrowed from a reminiscence collection or from someone's attic!
- Selection of grocery replicas (from toy-stores)
- Photographs of local scenes - then and now; old postcards of the area
- Large map of the country
- Famous faces photographs
- Polaroid camera or digital camera and printer
- Trivia quiz books
- Dominoes, playing cards, bingo
- Local expertise and knowledge to get resources and information for sessions.

Note: for some sessions multiple copies of materials are required. Access to a colour photocopier and to a laminator can help in preparing these.

Monitoring progress of maintenance sessions

It is important to keep a session-by-session record of each member's response to and involvement in the sessions, to enable you to adapt and plan the programme for future sessions. Photocopy the page opposite to keep a record of the whole group programme.

MAINTENANCE CST PROGRAMME

Monitoring progress form

NAMES OF MEMBERS	ATTENDED? YES/NO	INTEREST	COMMUNICATION	ENJOYMENT	MOOD
1.					
2.					
3.					
4.					
5.					
6.					
7.					
8.					

Rate each area in relation to today's session with a number from 1 to 5 as follows (use 2s and 4s to reflect ratings in between the descriptions given:

Interest: 1 = No interest; 2 = Little interest shown; 3 = Some interest shown
                       4 = Interest shown; 5 = Great interest shown

Communication: 1 = No communication; 2 = Little communication; 3 = Some response
                       4 = Communicates well; 5 = Communicates very well

Enjoyment: 1 = Does not show enjoyment of the session today;
                       2 = Very little enjoyment today; 3 = Some enjoyment shown;
                       4 = Enjoys the session; 5 = Enjoys the session greatly

Mood: 1 = In very low mood today, appears depressed or anxious;
                       2 = Low mood today; 3 = Some signs of good mood;
                       4 = General good mood today;
                       5 = Very good mood, appears happy and relaxed today

Session theme:

Activities used today:

Comments:

THIS PAGE CAN BE PHOTOCOPIED

Making a difference 2

Guidance for co-facilitators of cognitive stimulation therapy

Recommended preparation:

- Take the time to have a brief look at what the upcoming session is. This gives you the opportunity to put forward any suggestions that you may feel could work in the session
- Before the session take the time to remind each attendee what is going to be happening so that they can prepare themselves for it, and remind them what the session will be focusing on
- Try to arrive promptly so that no attendee is left waiting for a prolonged period of time for the group to start.

What is expected from the co-facilitator?

- It is important to be bright, positive and bubbly as this will have a direct effect on the attendees of the session
- Take the song sheet and newspaper off the attendees after the initial activity in order to give them the best chance of engaging with the main activity and with others
- If the person leading the group asks for help, let the attendees of the session help as much as possible
- If there are any silences, for example when the group leader is giving out materials for that session, unless one of the attendees is talking, see it as time to engage with the residents/attendees on a related topic to the session
- At the same time, even if there may appear to be a pause, allow time for the attendees to talk and answer for themselves
- Try to engage with all the attendees and encourage interaction between the members
- Try to keep the conversation as a group rather than subgroups. If you feel someone has something interesting to say you can always come back to it
- Although interaction and opinion is encouraged from yourself, it is important to remember that the focus of the group is the people who are attending and the input/opinions they provide
- It is important to remember and recognise that any opinion is valid and should be regarded as legitimate even if it is known to be an incorrect response/answer. Try not to correct the person.

Maintenance CST sessions

SESSION ONE | # My life (life history)

Your ideas

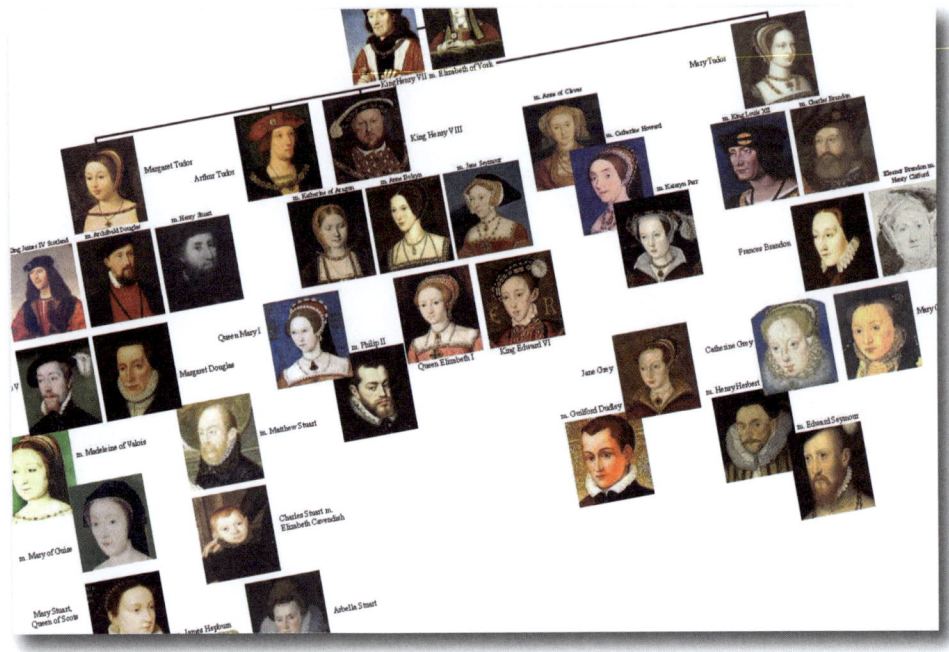

Opening (10 minutes)

❏ All members individually welcomed to the group by name
❏ On the first maintenance session as a group, discuss a name for the group – write the name on the whiteboard, and have a discussion about whether to continue using the name you've previously used for your CST groups or changing the name for this further 24 weeks. It is useful to have a vote; following which write the winning name prominently on the board
❏ As a group, sing together the group's 'theme song', led by song leader (use song book or CD)
❏ Discuss day, month, year, season, weather, time, name and address of the place you are in (use whiteboard)
❏ Discuss something currently in the news (use a newspaper, magazine or photograph).

Warm up

❏ Play a soft-ball game for a few minutes – when throwing the ball, people may either state their own name, or, for the more able, the name of the person they are throwing the ball to. As the main activity is going to be 'my life and personal diaries' ask members to say the origin/meaning of their name or surname.

Main activity (25 to 30 minutes)

Your ideas

Suggested activities:
- Ask members to fill out a printed sheet asking their name, father's name, mother's name, schools attended (etc) to form the first page of a memory diary
- Ask members to draw a family tree, including names and surnames of their family. You can show examples from the royal family as visual stimuli. Ask members to discuss the family tree shown with faces from Henry VIII's family tree and generate discussion about their opinions about the different marriages, wives, and so on.
- Ask members to talk about peculiarities in their family like the favourite relative or black sheep of the family and/or discuss the origin of their name and or surname. Have you been named after someone? A saint, family friend, relative?
- Talk about the meaning of surnames, you can find a complete definition of surnames, origins and meanings on the internet http://www.surnamedb.com/. Ask members to discuss whether or not they can link themselves with the meaning of their surname
- When known, ask participants to talk about characteristics of the place where their surname comes from and establish links between those objects and their personality, likes and dislikes.

Triggers

- Family trees
- Surnames information
- Life history sheet.

Closing (10 to 15 minutes)

❏ Thank everyone individually for attending and contributing to the session
❏ Summarise the discussion and ideas raised – seek feedback
❏ Sing theme song again
❏ Reminder of time and content of next session and farewells.

SESSION TWO | # Current affairs

Your ideas

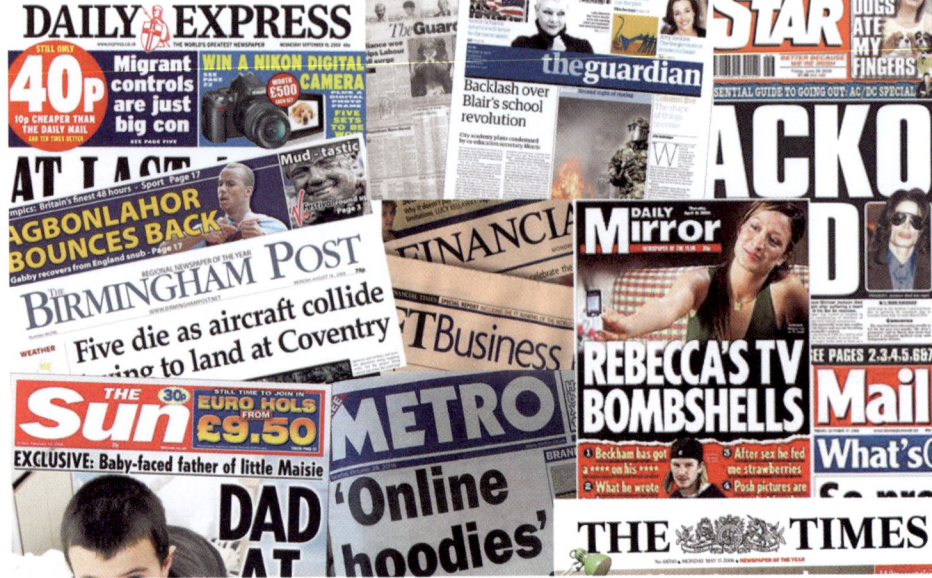

Opening (10 minutes)

❏ All members individually welcomed to the group by name
❏ Draw attention to the name of the group (on the whiteboard)
❏ Remind everyone of the activity in the last session
❏ As a group, sing together the group's 'theme song', led by song leader (use song book or CD)
❏ Discuss day, month, year, season, weather, time, name and address of the place you are in (use whiteboard)
❏ Discuss something currently in the news (use a newspaper, magazine or photograph).

Warm up

❏ Play a soft-ball game for a few minutes – when throwing the ball, people may either state their own name, or, for the more able, the name of the person they are throwing the ball to. As the main activity is going to be 'current affairs' ask members to select from a list of selected newspapers and magazines (with printed logos) the one they prefer, and why, when throwing the ball.

Start session by asking members about anything they've seen recently in the news.

Main activity (25 to 30 minutes)

Suggested activities:
- Discuss issues from a selection of recent magazines, special supplements, local newspapers and picture magazines. Have multiple copies of interesting articles (laminated if possible), so everyone has the same piece to look at

Making a difference **2**

- Use cue cards to evoke conversation on news, views, attitudes, dreams and aspirations. "What do you think of…?" Further examples are given below
- Compare a current news topic with one from a newspaper from the 40s/50s/60s/70s. You can find old articles on the archive from The Times. Discuss differences between them
- If possible, using a wireless laptop and data projector, present interactive news (e.g. Sky news, BBC news) to the group and generate discussion about it
- Discuss local topics, rubbish collection, green spaces, parking permits from the local area, newsletters, magazines
- Play the Room 101 ideas game. Invite participants to discuss their dislikes in relation to a current news article. Participants have to choose the item they dislike from a presented current new category (e.g. famous celebrities, type of food) and explain the reasons behind it. Any item can go in the room 101 and it is also possible for an item to be nominated more than once.

Triggers

- Newspapers
- Newspaper archive news
- Magazines
- Local newsletters, magazines
- Wireless laptop
- Data projector.

Current affairs including topics and possible comparisons with old news (some suggestions to build on!):
- DISCOVERY & TECHNOLOGY: first time man went to the moon
- POLITICS: first woman to become prime minister
- WAR: end of the Second World War and Hitler's death
- ROYAL FAMILY: first born child for the Queen

Current affairs questions (some suggestions to build on!):
- Should men and women have different roles – should men do the cooking, cleaning and laundry?
- What do you think of today's fashion?
- What do you think of same-sex weddings?
- What do you think about women putting up shelves or mending the car?
- What's your opinion in relation to the Royal Family? Would we be better off without them?
- What's your favourite charity?
- Who in the world do you admire the most?
- Where is your favourite place in the world?
- Are mobile phones a good thing? Do you have one or would like one? Does anyone in your family have one? (Demonstrate if necessary)
- Should there be a retirement age for everyone? What should it be?
- Is it too easy now to get a divorce?

Closing (10 to 15 minutes)

- ❏ Thank everyone individually for attending and contributing to the session
- ❏ Summarise the discussion and ideas raised – seek feedback
- ❏ Sing theme song again
- ❏ Reminder of time and content of next session
- ❏ Farewells.

SESSION THREE | **Food**

Your ideas

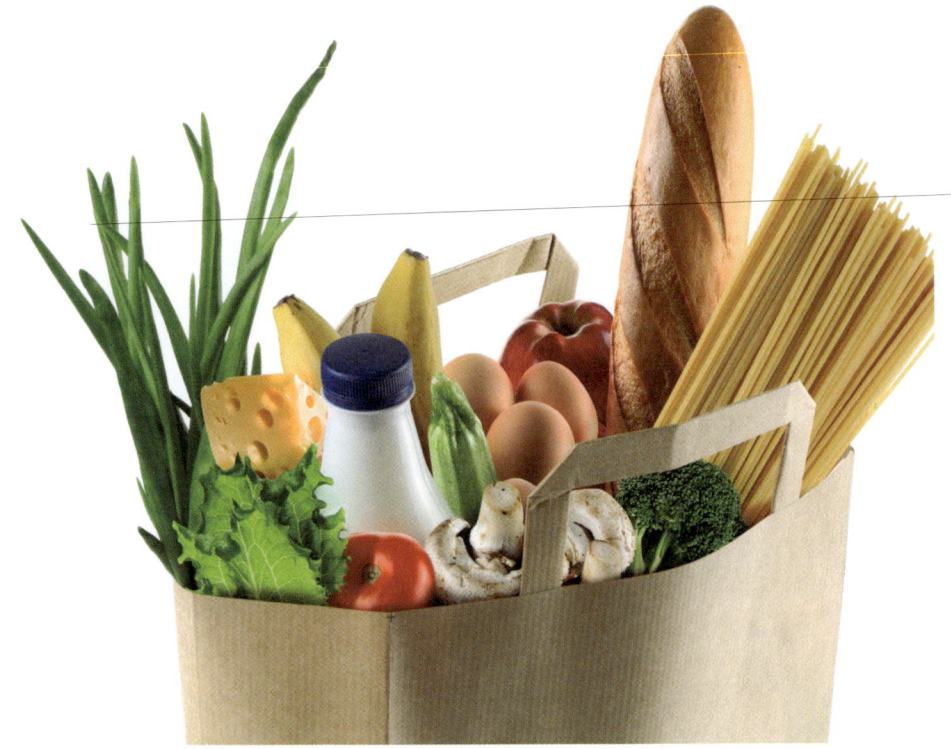

Opening (10 minutes)

❏ All members individually welcomed to the group by name
❏ Draw attention to the name of the group (on the whiteboard)
❏ Remind everyone of the activity in the last session. As a group, sing together the group's 'theme song', led by song leader (use song book or CD)
❏ Discuss day, month, year, season, weather, time, name and address of the place you are in (use whiteboard)
❏ Discuss something currently in the news (use a newspaper, magazine or photograph).

Warm up

❏ Play a soft-ball game for a few minutes – when throwing the ball, people may either state their own name, or, for the more able, the name of the person they are throwing the ball to. As the main activity is going to be 'food' ask members to say their favourite food or any food they particularly dislike, when catching the ball.

MAINTENANCE CST SESSIONS

Main activity (25 to 30 minutes)

Your ideas

Suggested activities:
- Taste foods which act as memory triggers or have personal meaning e.g. cream soda, ginger beer, bread pudding, spices, Bovril. Adapt to group participants
- Brainstorm food categories on the whiteboard, listing as many as possible in each category (e.g. soups, meats, puddings, fish, vegetables)
- Complete names of food items e.g. Yorkshire X; Bakewell X; self-raising X; and /or name a food beginning with a particular letter
- Using real groceries (preferable) or miniature grocery replicas which have been priced, give people a budget and a scenario to plan, e.g. a dinner for four, a Christmas dinner for six
- Using real groceries (preferable) or miniature grocery replicas categorise the foods, e.g. for different mealtimes, special occasions, savoury / sweet
- Present a selection of different food categories from country of origin plus cards or groceries e.g. Indian, Chinese, Italian, British, Greek. Ask participants to discuss them and organise them into the different categories. Encourage participants to talk about their favourite food and seek opinions about the different meals.

Triggers

- Food groceries
- Board
- List of food items.

Closing (10 to 15 minutes)

❑ Thank everyone individually for attending and contributing to the session
❑ Summarise the discussion and ideas raised – seek feedback
❑ Sing theme song again
❑ Reminder of time and content of next session
❑ Farewells.

Making a difference 2

SESSION FOUR | **Being creative**

Your ideas

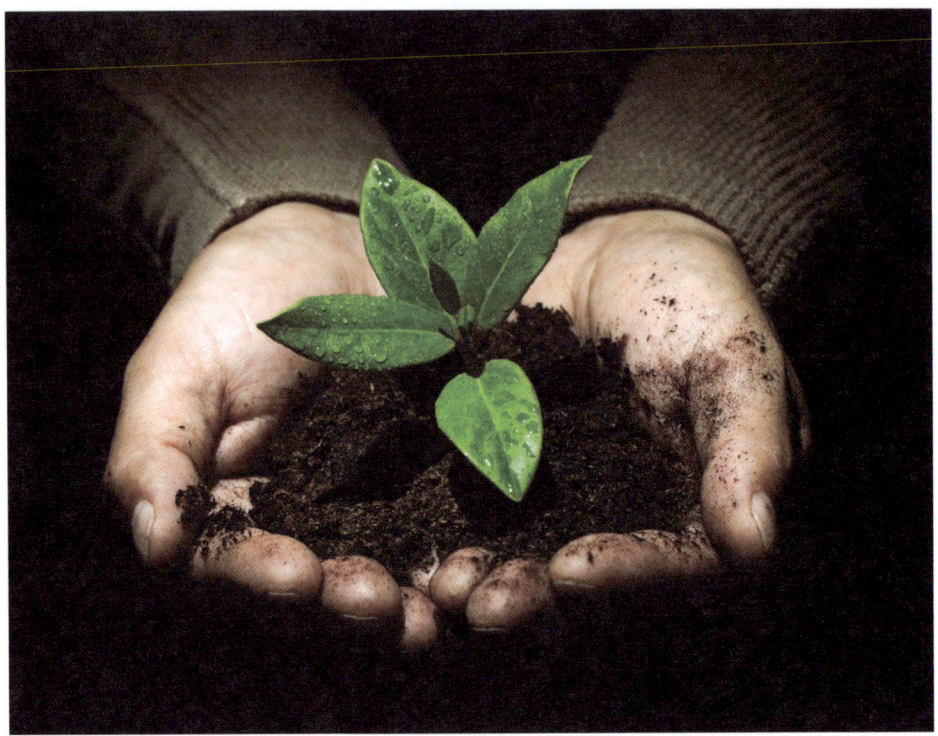

Opening (10 minutes)

- All members individually welcomed to the group by name
- Draw attention to the name of the group (on the whiteboard)
- Remind everyone of the activity in the last session. As a group, sing together the group's 'theme song', led by song leader (use song book or CD)
- Discuss day, month, year, season, weather, time, name and address of the place you are in (use whiteboard)
- Discuss something currently in the news (use a newspaper, magazine or photograph).

Warm up

- Play a soft-ball game for a few minutes – when throwing the ball, people may either state their own name, or, for the more able, the name of the person they are throwing the ball to. As the main activity is going to be 'creativity' ask members to say their favourite colour or favourite flower and, if known, the reason for their choice.

MAINTENANCE CST SESSIONS

Main activity (25 to 30 minutes)

Your ideas

Suggested activities:
- Cookery: Make an apple crumble, for example. Divide the task into multiple tasks so you can enable all to participate (e.g. greasing bowl, mixing ingredients, making crumble mixture, peeling and slicing apples)
- Creating a seasonal collage: Use natural items and pictures to create a collage e.g. autumn leaves, spring flowers
- Making a group collage: Use magazine words, items and pictures to create a collage that group participants feel can represent the group
- Dream house/garden collage: Use catalogues and magazines for group participants to create a collage of their dream garden and/or house
- Clay modelling: Make animals or sculptures
- Gardening: Plant bulbs or seeds – check progress in future weeks
- Making wood figures.

Triggers

- Garden seeds, pots
- Collage materials
- Cooking materials
- Clay modelling materials
- Wood figures.

Closing (10 to 15 minutes)

- ❏ Thank everyone individually for attending and contributing to the session
- ❏ Summarise the discussion and ideas raised – seek feedback
- ❏ Sing theme song again
- ❏ Reminder of time and content of next session
- ❏ Farewells.

SESSION FIVE | **Number games**

Your ideas

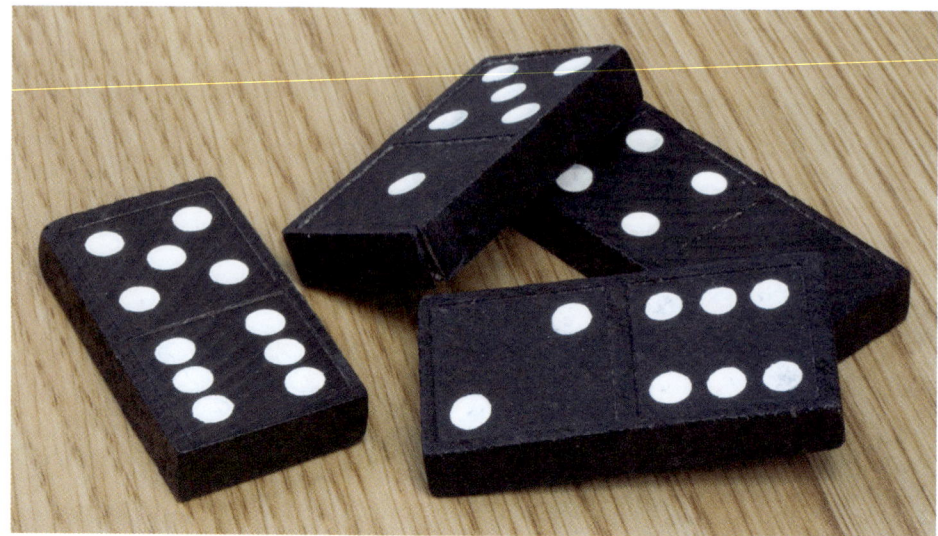

Opening (10 minutes)

❏ All members individually welcomed to the group by name
❏ Draw attention to the name of the group (on the whiteboard)
❏ Remind everyone of the activity in the last session. As a group, sing together the group's 'theme song', led by song leader (use song book or CD)
❏ Discuss day, month, year, season, weather, time, name and address of the place you are in (use whiteboard)
❏ Discuss something currently in the news (use a newspaper, magazine or photograph).

Warm up

❏ Play a soft-ball game for a few minutes – when throwing the ball, people may either state their own name, or, for the more able, the name of the person they are throwing the ball to. As the main activity is going to be 'number games' ask members to say any favourite or special number they've got, e.g. "22 as it is the day I was married"; "7 as it is my lucky number".

Main activity (25 to 30 minutes)

Your ideas

Suggested activities:
- Games involving the recognition and use of numbers e.g. bingo, dominoes, bendomino (a new type of dominos that includes the use of visuo-spatial abilities)
- Play 'snap' with playing cards. Or go around the group drawing the next card off a pack of cards, guessing whether it will be higher or lower than the previous card
- Guess how many items there are in a container (e.g. pennies in a small jar) – count them out to check whose guess is closest!
- A group game to guess how many items (e.g. pennies, beans) there are. Each participant chooses to hide 0 to 3 items in their hand. Everyone in the group has to guess how many items there are in total in the group. After everyone has expressed their thoughts, participants have to open their hands and the items are counted. The participant wins who has the closest guess to the total number of items in the group.
- Play perudo, a classic ancient Peruvian dice game where each player has a cup and five dice of the same colour. A process of bidding, bluffing and luck reduces the number of dice in play.

Triggers

- Cards
- Bingo set
- Number games
- Small items (pennies, beans).

Closing (10 to 15 minutes)

❏ Thank everyone individually for attending and contributing to the session
❏ Summarise the discussion and ideas raised – seek feedback
❏ Sing theme song again
❏ Reminder of time and content of next session
❏ Farewells.

SESSION SIX | # Team games/quiz

Your ideas

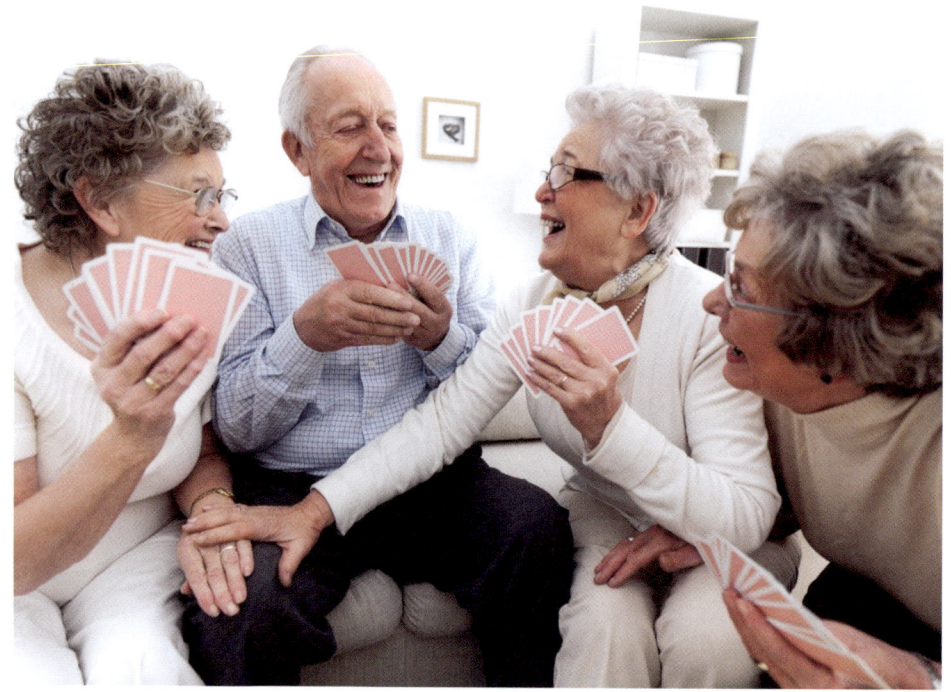

Opening (10 minutes)

❏ All members individually welcomed to the group by name
❏ Draw attention to the name of the group (on the whiteboard)
❏ Remind everyone of the activity in the last session. As a group, sing together the group's 'theme song', led by song leader (use song book or CD)
❏ Discuss day, month, year, season, weather, time, name and address of the place you are in (use whiteboard)
❏ Discuss something currently in the news (use a newspaper, magazine or photograph).

Warm up

❏ Play soft-ball game for a few minutes – when throwing the ball, people may either state their own name, or, for the more able, the name of the person they are throwing the ball to. As the main activity is going to be a 'quiz' ask members to say their favourite subject when doing a quiz or a subject they think they are very good at. Give examples depending on the group, using cards as aids if necessary e.g. history, nature, celebrities.

MAINTENANCE CST SESSIONS

Main activity (25 to 30 minutes)

Your ideas

Suggested activities:
- Team games: divide the group into two teams, ask them to choose a team name, and play trivial quiz, music quiz or similar. Give prizes to the entire group. Have a special group tea with cakes, special treats etc.

Triggers

- Quiz book
- Quiz cards
- Calculation board
- Music quiz CD
- Music MP3 player, speakers
- Laptop.

Closing (10 to 15 minutes)

❏ Thank everyone individually for attending and contributing to the session
❏ Summarise the discussion and ideas raised – seek feedback
❏ Sing theme song again
❏ Reminder of time and content of next session
❏ Farewells.

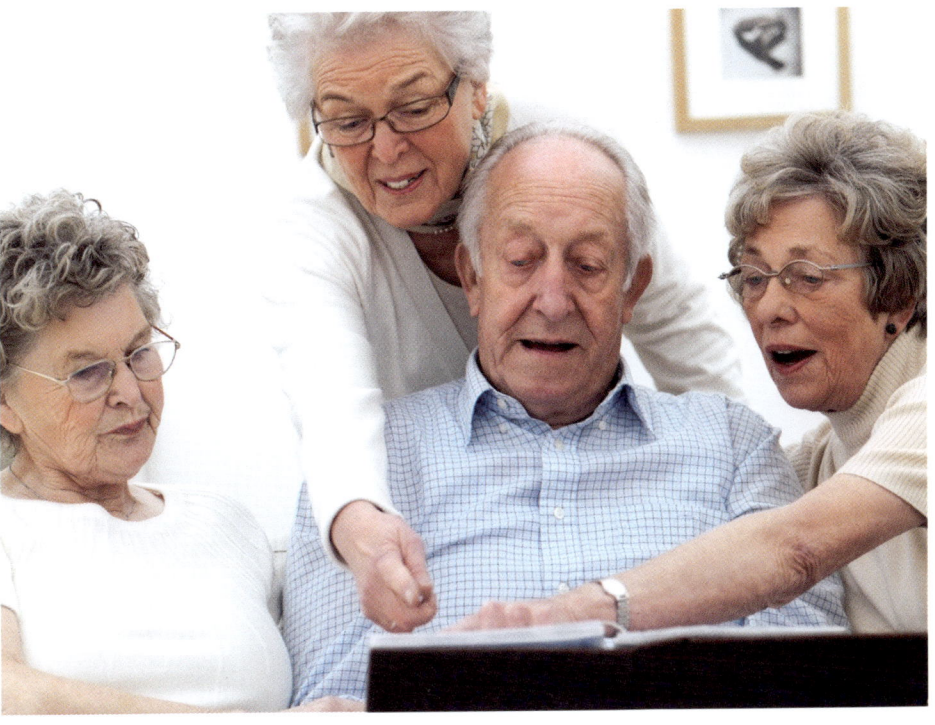

Making a difference 2

SESSION SEVEN | Sound

Your ideas

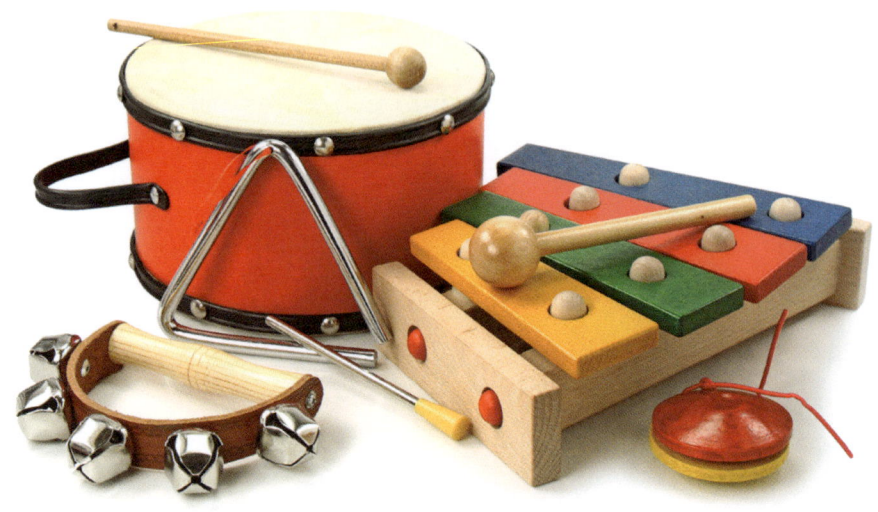

Opening (10 minutes)

❏ All members individually welcomed to the group by name
❏ Draw attention to the name of the group (on the whiteboard)
❏ Remind everyone of the activity in the last session. As a group, sing together the group's 'theme song', led by song leader (use song book or CD)
❏ Discuss day, month, year, season, weather, time, name and address of the place you are in (use whiteboard)
❏ Discuss something currently in the news (use a newspaper, magazine or photograph).

Warm up

❏ Play a soft-ball game for a few minutes – when throwing the ball, people may either state their own name, or, for the more able, the name of the person they are throwing the ball to. As the main activity is going to be 'sounds' ask members to say their favourite song or instrument or type of music.

Main activity (25 to 30 minutes)

Your ideas

Suggested activities:
- Percussion instruments can be given to each person in the group, so they can be played with familiar music (such as popular 1940's, 1950's music)
- Play selected tracks from a compilation music CD from the appropriate era – members are invited to name the song or singer; if necessary, provide a choice of two or three on the whiteboard as members listen to the song
- Sound effects CDs, which include different categories, such as 'indoor sounds' and 'outdoor sounds' (e.g. animal noises), to be matched with the correct picture. This provides people with both visual and auditory stimulation, making the task easier.
- Play a musical bingo game that can be found at www.speechmark.com or you can create your own.

Triggers

- Instruments
- Music CDs
- Sound CDs
- Pictures or objects
- Musical bingo game.

Closing (10 to 15 minutes)

❏ Thank everyone individually for attending and contributing to the session
❏ Summarise the discussion and ideas raised – seek feedback
❏ Sing theme song again
❏ Reminder of time and content of next session
❏ Farewells.

SESSION EIGHT | Physical games

Your ideas

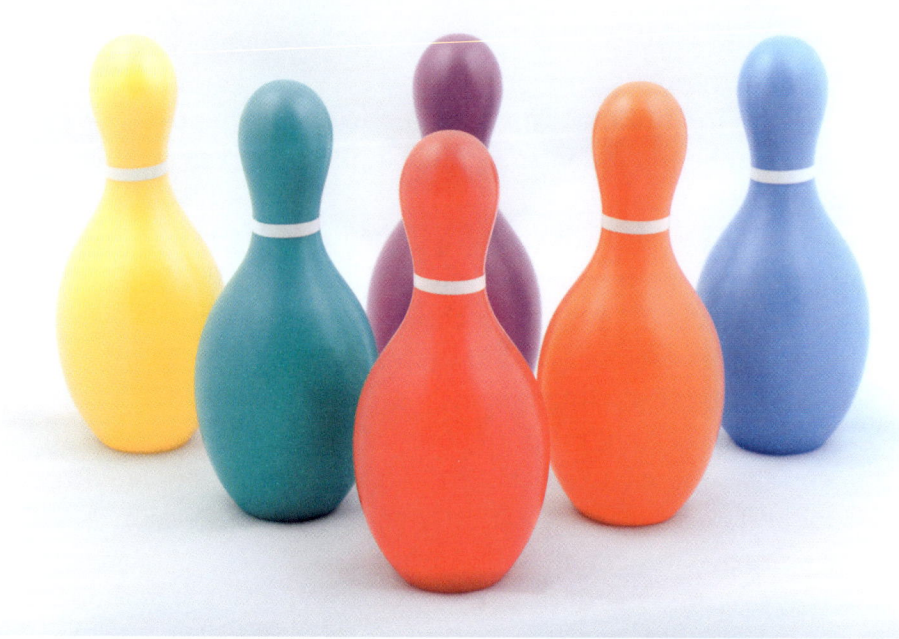

Opening (10 minutes)

❏ All members individually welcomed to the group by name
❏ Draw attention to the name of the group (on the whiteboard)
❏ Remind everyone of the activity in the last session. As a group, sing together the group's 'theme song', led by song leader (use song book or CD)
❏ Discuss day, month, year, season, weather, time, name and address of the place you are in (use whiteboard)
❏ Discuss something currently in the news (use a newspaper, magazine or photograph).

Warm up

❏ Play a soft-ball game for a few minutes – when throwing the ball, people may either state their own name, or, for the more able, the name of the person they are throwing the ball to. As the main activity is going to be 'physical games' ask members to say their favourite physical game, use card aids if needed
❏ Throw a soft ball around, asking people to say something about themselves as they catch the ball; e.g. their name, where they come from, their former occupation, favourite food, favourite colour.

MAINTENANCE CST SESSIONS

Main activity (25 to 30 minutes)

Your ideas

Suggested activities:
- Physical game, such as skittles or indoor bowls or boules, dart ball game, activity rings, floor basketball which involves teamwork, or any other game that involves physical activity and the group would enjoy
- Play seatwork with music from the Winslow catalogue
- Play parachute in the group trying to insert the ball in the middle.

Triggers

- Physical games
- Calculation board
- Soft ball
- Favourite categories cards.

Closing (10 to 15 minutes)

❏ Thank everyone individually for attending and contributing to the session
❏ Summarise the discussion and ideas raised – seek feedback
❏ Sing theme song again
❏ Reminder of time and content of next session
❏ Farewells.

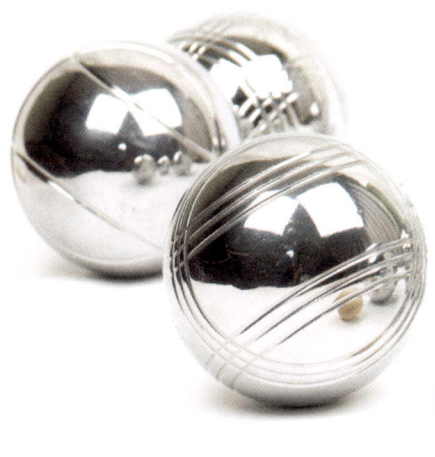
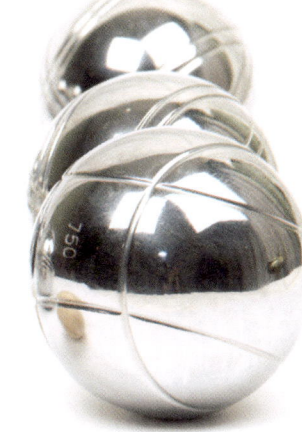

SESSION NINE | # Categorising objects

Your ideas

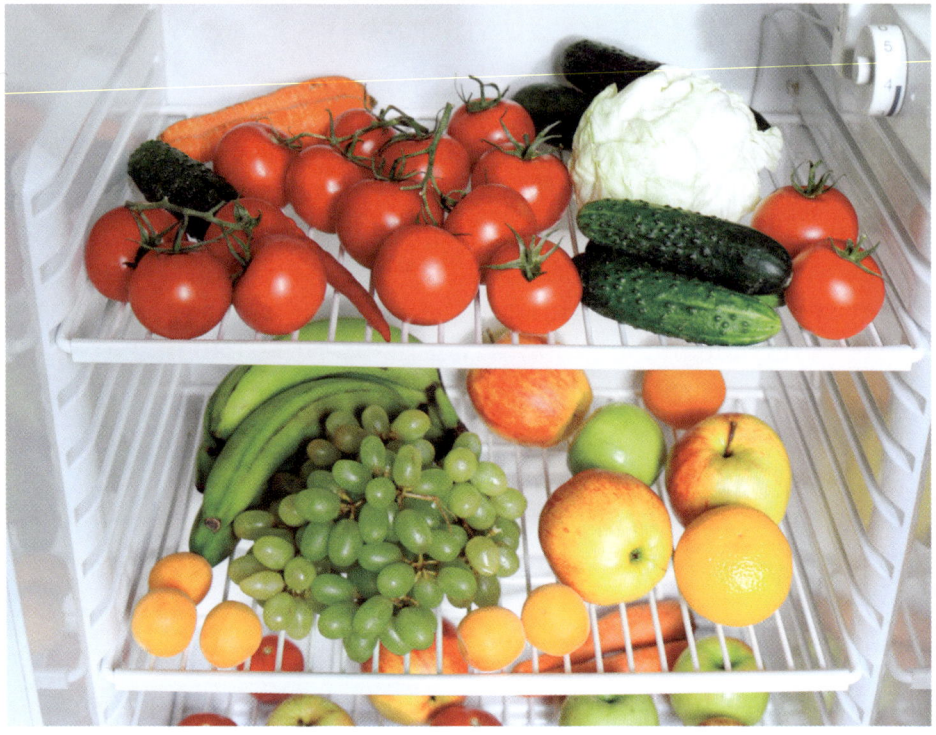

Opening (10 minutes)

- All members individually welcomed to the group by name
- Draw attention to the name of the group (on the whiteboard)
- Remind everyone of the activity in the last session. As a group, sing together the group's 'theme song', led by song leader (use song book or CD)
- Discuss day, month, year, season, weather, time, name and address of the place you are in (use whiteboard)
- Discuss something currently in the news (use a newspaper, magazine or photograph).

Warm up

- Play a soft-ball game for a few minutes – when throwing the ball, people may either state their own name, or, for the more able, the name of the person they are throwing the ball to. Ask participants to say their favourite month of the year or season or weather.

MAINTENANCE CST SESSIONS

Main activity (25 to 30 minutes)

Your ideas

Suggested activities:
- Ask people to think of words beginning with a particular letter in a particular category, either picked from a card or from a list (see list below) e.g. countries, boys' names, girls' names, a vegetable, a flower, an alcoholic drink, something at Christmas
- Write the category on the board, and the task is to think of as many examples as possible
- Have 20 or so objects, or coloured pictures of objects, on the table; the group's task is to group them in different ways: for example, by use, colour, and/or initial letter
- Play the odd man out game; which of three objects is the odd one out?

Triggers

- Coloured pictures of objects
- Real objects, different fruits, clothes, etc
- White board
- Letter aid rule.

Closing (10 to 15 minutes)

❏ Thank everyone individually for attending and contributing to the session
❏ Summarise the discussion and ideas raised – seek feedback
❏ Sing theme song again
❏ Reminder of time and content of next session
❏ Farewells.

Suggestions of possible categories

1. Countries
2. Boys' names
3. Girls' names
4. Vegetables
5. Flowers
6. Alcoholic drinks
7. Something at Christmas
8. Famous singers
9. Foods
10. Towns / cities
11. World leaders (past and present)
12. Animals
13. Birds
14. Films
15. Songs
16. Things found in the supermarket
17. Things found in the kitchen
18. Things found in the shed
19. Things found in the garden
20. Musical instrument
21. Fish
22. Colour
23. Item of clothing
24. Means of transport
25. Something you fear
26. Something you enjoy
27. Film star
28. TV programme
29. Sport
30. Counties / states.

Making a difference 2

SESSION TEN | # Household treasures

Your ideas

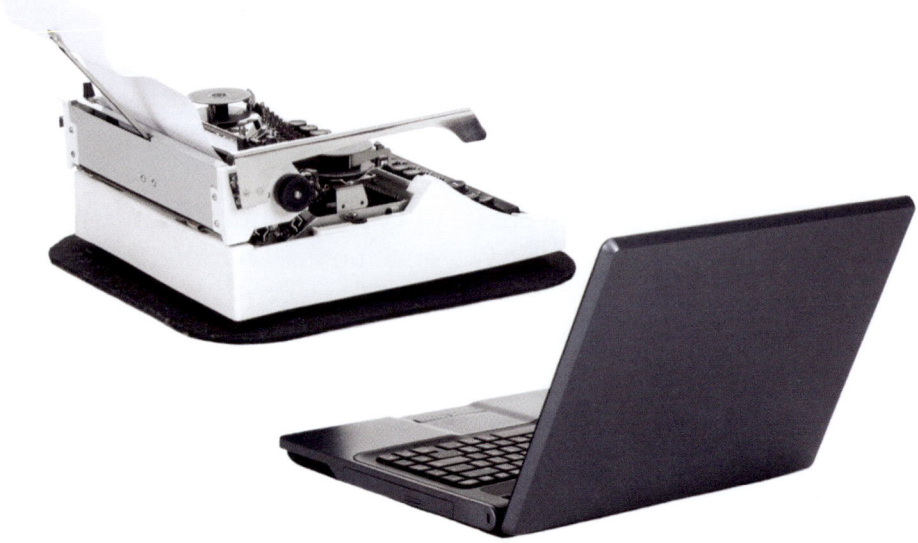

Opening (10 minutes)

❏ All members individually welcomed to the group by name
❏ Draw attention to the name of the group (on the whiteboard)
❏ Remind everyone of the activity in the last session. As a group, sing together the group's 'theme song', led by song leader (use song book or CD)
❏ Discuss day, month, year, season, weather, time, name and address of the place you are in (use whiteboard)
❏ Discuss something currently in the news (use a newspaper, magazine or photograph).

Warm up

❏ Play a soft-ball game for a few minutes – when throwing the ball, people may either state their own name, or, for the more able, the name of the person they are throwing the ball to. As the main activity is going to be 'household treasures', ask members to say their favourite, special, oldest or newest object they have at home, e.g. their mum's engagement ring, the kettle and so on.

Main activity (25 to 30 minutes)

Your ideas

Suggested activities:
- Present old and new objects to the group (old telephone and mobile phone, old iron and new iron, old kettle and new kettle, old keys and new keys, old typewriter and new computer, old records and new mp3 player, old milk bottles and new milk containers). Ask participants to match them and give a demonstration of how to use them. Generate discussion about the objects
- You can also look for differences and similarities between the new and old objects
- Ask about likes and dislikes amongst the group between the new and old versions. For example, "In your opinion, which one do you think is the best? The one that looks better? The most useful one? The one you prefer?".

Triggers

- Selection of old and new objects
- Household treasures pictures and objects
- Old objects can be found through the Winslow catalogue or a reminiscence box.

Closing (10 to 15 minutes)

❏ Thank everyone individually for attending and contributing to the session
❏ Summarise the discussion and ideas raised – seek feedback
❏ Sing theme song again
❏ Reminder of time and content of next session
❏ Farewells.

SESSION ELEVEN | # Useful tips (house)

Your ideas

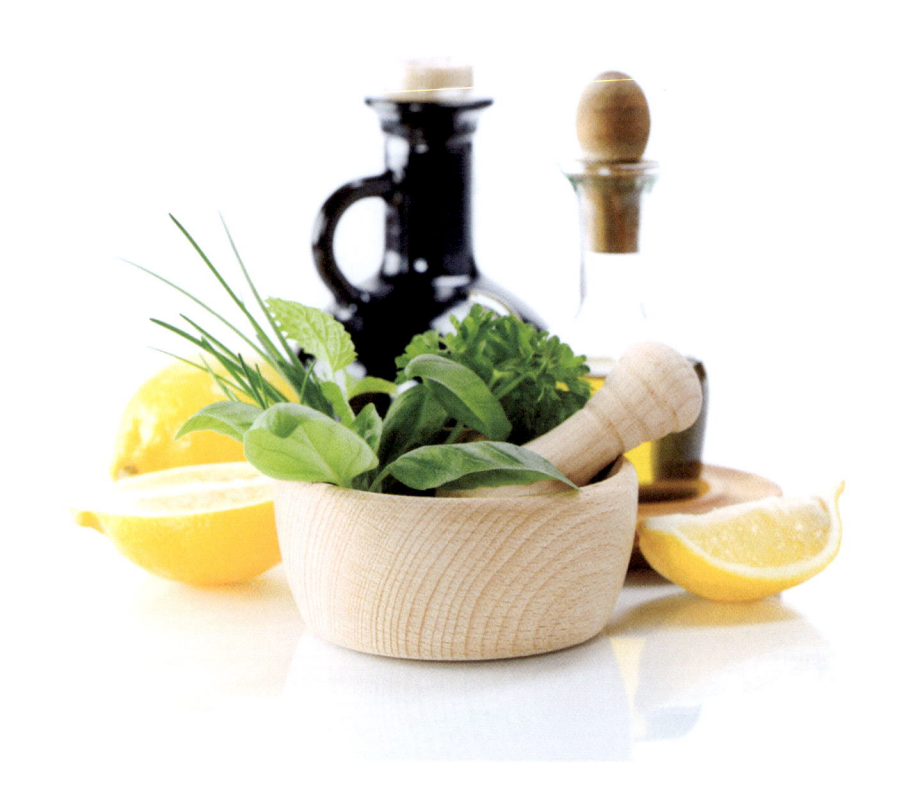

Opening (10 minutes)

- ❏ All members individually welcomed to the group by name
- ❏ Draw attention to the name of the group (on the whiteboard)
- ❏ Remind everyone of the activity in the last session. As a group, sing together the group's 'theme song', led by song leader (use song book or CD)
- ❏ Discuss day, month, year, season, weather, time, name and address of the place you are in (use whiteboard)
- ❏ Discuss something currently in the news (use a newspaper, magazine or photograph).

Warm up

- ❏ Play a soft-ball game for a few minutes – when throwing the ball, people may either state their own name, or, for the more able, the name of the person they are throwing the ball to. As the main activity is going to be 'useful tips' ask members to say the best/most useful tip or advice someone has ever told him/her.

Main activity (25 to 30 minutes)

Your ideas

Suggested activities:
- Using information from a book about customs and remedies from the past, encourage general discussion and ask participants how:
  - to soothe burns
  - to keep the milk fresh
  - to control pests
  - to care for pets
  - to care for flowers
  - to care for clothes
  - to suggest traditional decorating tips
  - to get a child to sleep.
- Ask participants to compare the old remedies with the new 'systems'. Ask opinion as to whether nowadays the type of household problem shown above can be solved quicker or more cheaply or more efficiently?
- Ask for opinions about where young people should look for advice about solving these problems now? Did people learn to solve these problems at school and/or home previously?

Triggers

- Hints and Tips book by Linda Gray: www.amazon.co.uk
- Good Housekeeping online: www.allaboutyou.com/goodhousekeeping
- Traditional Remedies book by Linda Gray: www.amazon.co.uk
- Grandma's Household Hints And Tips: www.homemade-dessert-recipes.com/helpful-household-hints.html.

Closing (10 to 15 minutes)

- ❑ Thank everyone individually for attending and contributing to the session
- ❑ Summarise the discussion and ideas raised – seek feedback
- ❑ Sing theme song again
- ❑ Reminder of time and content of next session
- ❑ Farewells.

SESSION TWELVE | # Thinking cards

Your ideas

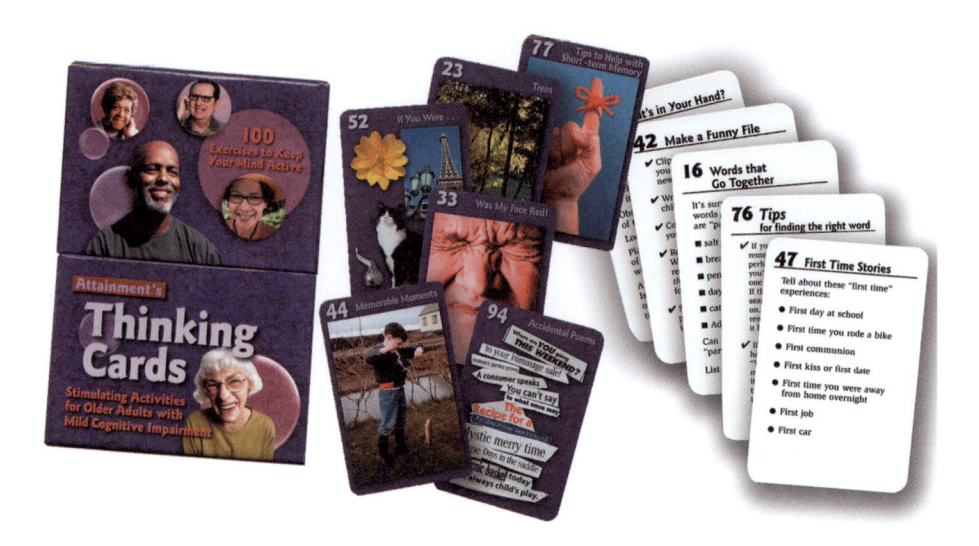

Opening (10 minutes)

- ❏ All members individually welcomed to the group by name
- ❏ Draw attention to the name of the group (on the whiteboard)
- ❏ Remind everyone of the activity in the last session. As a group, sing together the group's 'theme song', led by song leader (use song book or CD)
- ❏ Discuss day, month, year, season, weather, time, name and address of the place you are in (use whiteboard)
- ❏ Discuss something currently in the news (use a newspaper, magazine or photograph).

Warm up

- ❏ Play a soft-ball game for a few minutes – when throwing the ball, people may either state their own name, or, for the more able, the name of the person they are throwing the ball to. Ask members to say their favourite place in the world.

Main activity (25 to 30 minutes)

Suggested activities:
- Use thinking cards asking 'discussion-provoking questions' to the members of the group. Generate discussion and encourage self expression (e.g. "What is your favourite charity? How do you think older people are treated in society?")

- Use case scenario 'Imagine' cards to ask members of the group what they would do in given situations. Use a selection of objects that promote discussion and help conversation. For example, imagine that you just have moved to a new house and while cleaning you discover a strange panel you've never noticed before. When pushing the door you realise the wall opens up. What is it behind the door? What do you see? What do you do? Other examples include: what would you do if you find a mouse in your home?; or what would you do if a young person knocks on your door asking for money for a charity? Generate discussion among the group
- Use 'Intuit' cards to ask members of the group questions like:
  - Which place would you most like to visit? France, Africa, China, Alaska?
  - Which of the following would you most like to develop yourself? Cheerfulness, honesty, patience?
  - How do you most like to learn? Lectures, books, experience, films, radio?
- Use the help of passports, case and maps to generate discussion.

Triggers

- Create your own thinking cards
- Thinking cards from:
  -      www.disabilitytraining.com
  -      www.winslow-cat.com/thinking-cards.html

Your ideas

Closing (10 to 15 minutes)

❏ Thank everyone individually for attending and contributing to the session
❏ Summarise the discussion and ideas raised – seek feedback
❏ Sing theme song again
❏ Reminder of time and content of next session
❏ Farewells.

SESSION THIRTEEN

Visual clips discussion

Your ideas

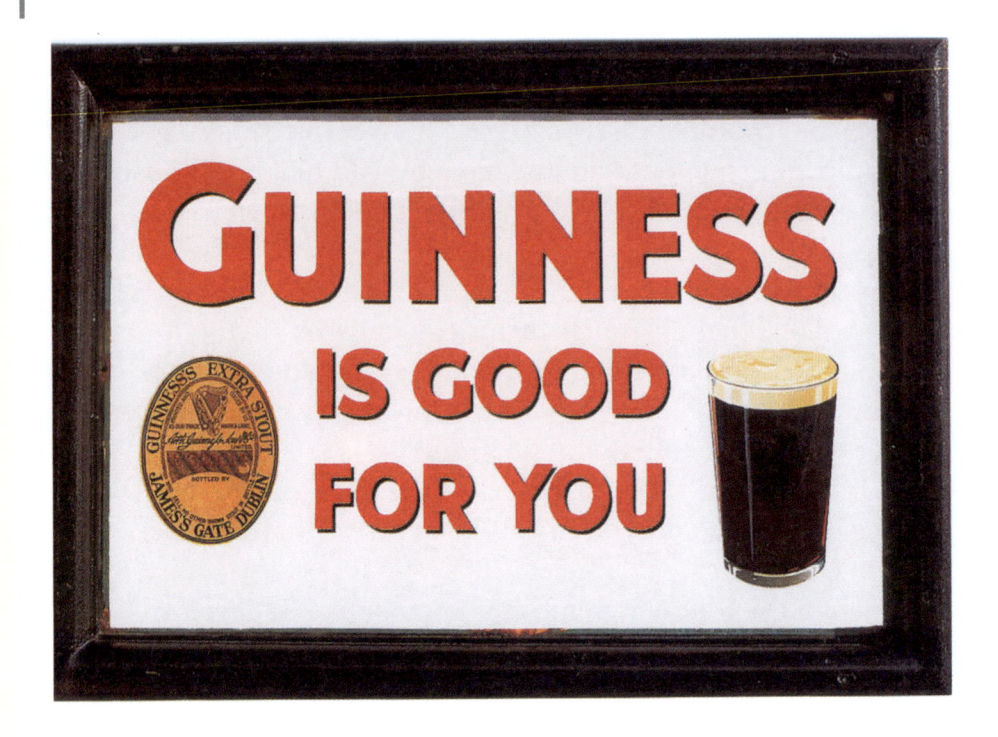

Opening (10 minutes)

❏ All members individually welcomed to the group by name
❏ Draw attention to the name of the group (on the whiteboard)
❏ Remind everyone of the activity in the last session. As a group, sing together the group's 'theme song', led by song leader (use song book or CD)
❏ Discuss day, month, year, season, weather, time, name and address of the place you are in (use whiteboard)
❏ Discuss something currently in the news (use a newspaper, magazine or photograph).

Warm up

❏ Play a soft-ball game for a few minutes – when throwing the ball, people may either state their own name, or, for the more able, the name of the person they are throwing the ball to. As the main activity is going to be 'slogans', present a selection of slogans (either from any of the Opie reminiscence books or ones downloaded from the internet) and ask about their favourite one.

MAINTENANCE CST SESSIONS

Main activity (25 to 30 minutes)

Suggested activities:
- Show participants a TV advertisement or play them theme tunes and ask them their opinion, what they think the presented tune or advertisement is about and to match products with the slogans used to advertise them
- Write five to ten slogans on a large sheet of paper. Hand out pictures of the products and have participants match each with the corresponding slogan
- Read a slogan and ask participants to call out the corresponding product
- Create a slogan. Ask individuals or whole groups to create their own slogan for a number of products. See if the rest of the group can guess the right product for each slogan
- Use large nostalgic advertising signs and postcards to present a product and match it with a new presentation of the same product. Generate discussion about how the presentation of the product has changed and if there are any differences or similarities. Ask them what they prefer about the new or old presentation.

Triggers
- TV advertisement (shown on TV or laptop)
- Sample slogans
- Advertisement from the past (Robert Opie collection).

Closing (10 to 15 minutes)

- ❏ Thank everyone individually for attending and contributing to the session
- ❏ Summarise the discussion and ideas raised – seek feedback
- ❏ Sing theme song again
- ❏ Reminder of time and content of next session
- ❏ Farewells.

Sample slogans

- "I liked the shaver so much, I bought the company", Remington shavers firm
- "The future's Orange"
- "Men can't help acting on Impulse"
- "Your Country Needs You", Lord Kitchener persuading millions of Britons to enlist for the First World War with the stirring poster
- "Labour isn't working", Margaret Thatcher comes into power in 1979
- "Good things come to those who wait", slogan created in the 1930s for brewer Guinness
- "Guinness is good for you"
- "Tingling fresh", the first television ad for Gibbs SR toothpaste
- "Snap, crackle and pop", Rice Krispies
- "Murray Mints, Murray Mints - too good to hurry mints"
- "Go to work on an egg", possibly the most famous catchphrase of the 1960s, transforming life for the Egg Marketing Board
- "Only the crumbliest, flakiest chocolate"
- "Shhh...you know who", Schweppes
- "Beanz meanz Heinz"
- "Refreshes the part other beers cannot reach", Heineken
- "Anytime, anyplace, anywhere", Martini
- "Naughty but nice", slogan for cream cakes
- "For mash get Smash", the TV debut of toy Martians advertising Cadbury's instant mashed potato in 1974
- "Is she or isn't she?", one of the earliest examples of sexual innuendo in advertising from Harmony Hairsprays
- "Just one Cornetto, give it to me - delicious ice cream, from Italy", many still find it difficult to hear Puccini without trilling the phrase.

Conversation starters

- What products have you bought because of the advertisement?
- What products would you never buy because of the advertisement?
- How do you decide which products to buy?
- Does advertising serve a useful purpose?
- What is your favourite slogan?
- Create a slogan to promote your talents
- Create a slogan for each month in the year
- Do you think that slogans are more effective on TV, over the radio, or in the newspaper?
- What is the oldest slogan you can remember?

Making a difference 2

SESSION FOURTEEN | **Art discussion**

Your ideas

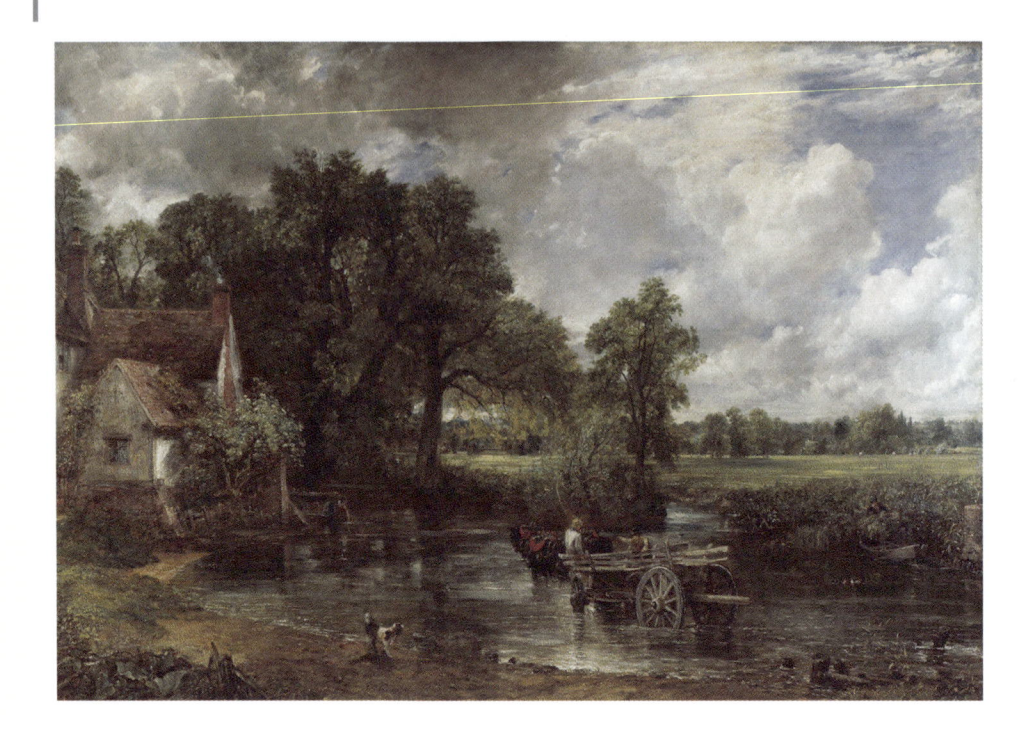

Opening (10 minutes)

❏ All members individually welcomed to the group by name
❏ Draw attention to the name of the group (on the whiteboard)
❏ Remind everyone of the activity in the last session. As a group, sing together the group's 'theme song', led by song leader (use song book or CD)
❏ Discuss day, month, year, season, weather, time, name and address of the place you are in (use whiteboard)
❏ Discuss something currently in the news (use a newspaper, magazine or photograph).

Warm up

❏ Play a soft-ball game for a few minutes – when throwing the ball, people may either state their own name, or, for the more able, the name of the person they are throwing the ball to. As the main activity is going to be 'art' ask members to choose from a selection of pictures the one they particularly like or dislike.

MAINTENANCE CST SESSIONS

Main activity (25 to 30 minutes)

Your ideas

Suggested activities:
- Present a selection of pictures of artworks ranging from classical to modern and ask participants what they think about them, their opinions of different types of art, colours they think might go together, whether they would have a particular presented piece of art in their house. Ask them what they can see, or what they think is going on, in the picture
- Ask participants to categorise art work into different categories e.g. modern, classic, abstract, white and black, colour
- Ask participants about their favourite painter/artist or artwork and share it with the group
- Ask participants what they think about the different types of art. Do they think modern art is a type of art?

Triggers

- Artwork pictures.

Closing (10 to 15 minutes)

❏ Thank everyone individually for attending and contributing to the session
❏ Summarise the discussion and ideas raised – seek feedback
❏ Sing theme song again
❏ Reminder of time and content of next session
❏ Farewells.

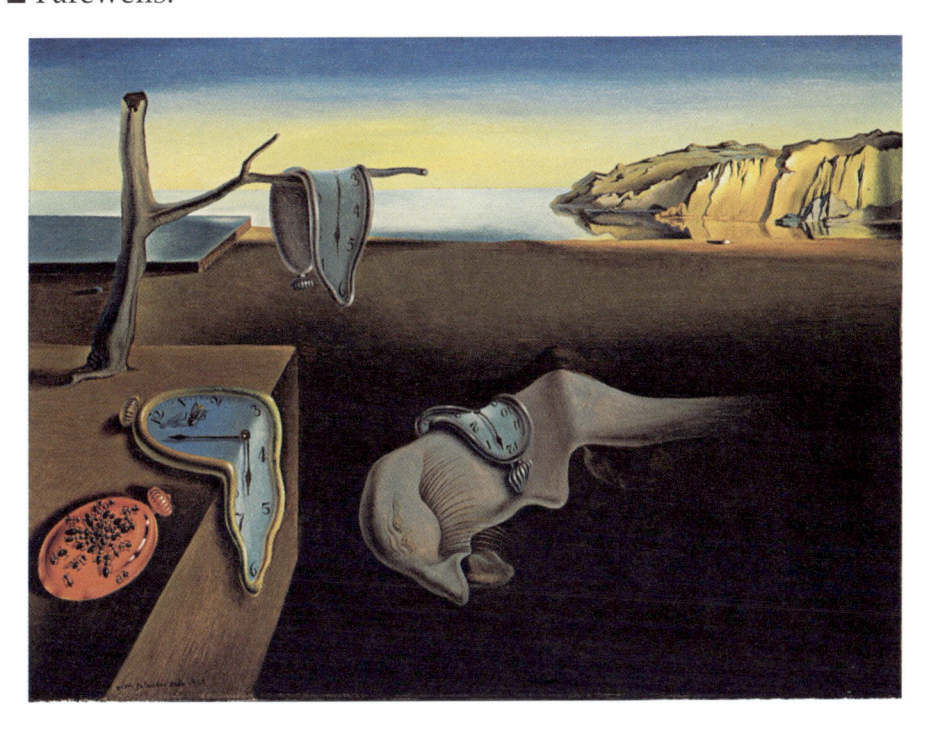

Making a difference 2

SESSION FIFTEEN | # Faces/scenes

Your ideas

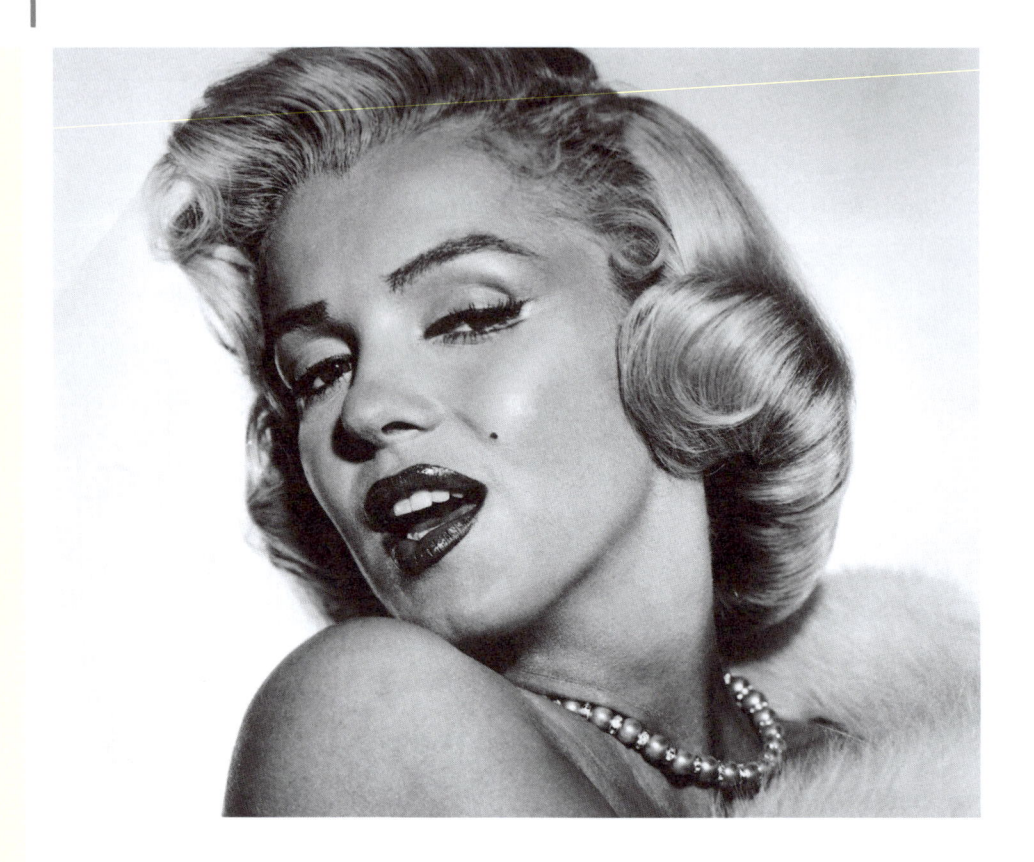

Opening (10 minutes)

- All members individually welcomed to the group by name
- Draw attention to the name of the group (on the whiteboard)
- Remind everyone of the activity in the last session. As a group, sing together the group's 'theme song', led by song leader (use song book or CD)
- Discuss day, month, year, season, weather, time, name and address of the place you are in (use whiteboard)
- Discuss something currently in the news (use a newspaper, magazine or photograph).

Warm up

- Play a soft-ball game for a few minutes – when throwing the ball, people may either state their own name, or, for the more able, the name of the person they are throwing the ball to. As the main activity is going to be 'famous faces' ask participants about their favourite famous actress/actor/singer.

MAINTENANCE CST SESSIONS

Main activity (25 to 30 minutes)

Your ideas

Suggested activities:
- Use multiple copies of laminated photographs of famous faces or of local scenes (e.g. from old postcards) so that everyone can look at the same picture. Give people one or more cards, and ask them their opinions about what they see, for example who is the most attractive, or oldest, or youngest? What do they have in common? How are they different? Which is the most peaceful place or most exciting place? Attempt to use opinions to generate memories for names of people, towns, cities, professions, and so on
- Use a Polaroid or digital camera and printer to generate photographs of group members and then match them with the real person.

Triggers

- Polaroid or digital camera
- Pictures of famous people or scenes.

Closing (10 to 15 minutes)

❏ Thank everyone individually for attending and contributing to the session
❏ Summarise the discussion and ideas raised – seek feedback
❏ Sing theme song again
❏ Reminder of time and content of next session
❏ Farewells.

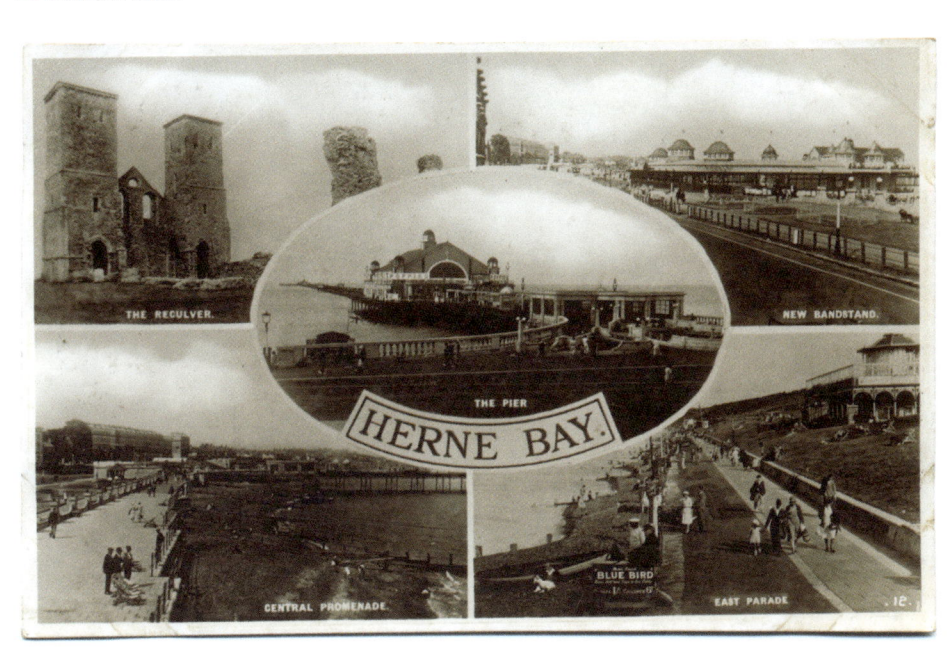

Making a difference 2

SESSION SIXTEEN | **Word game**

Your ideas

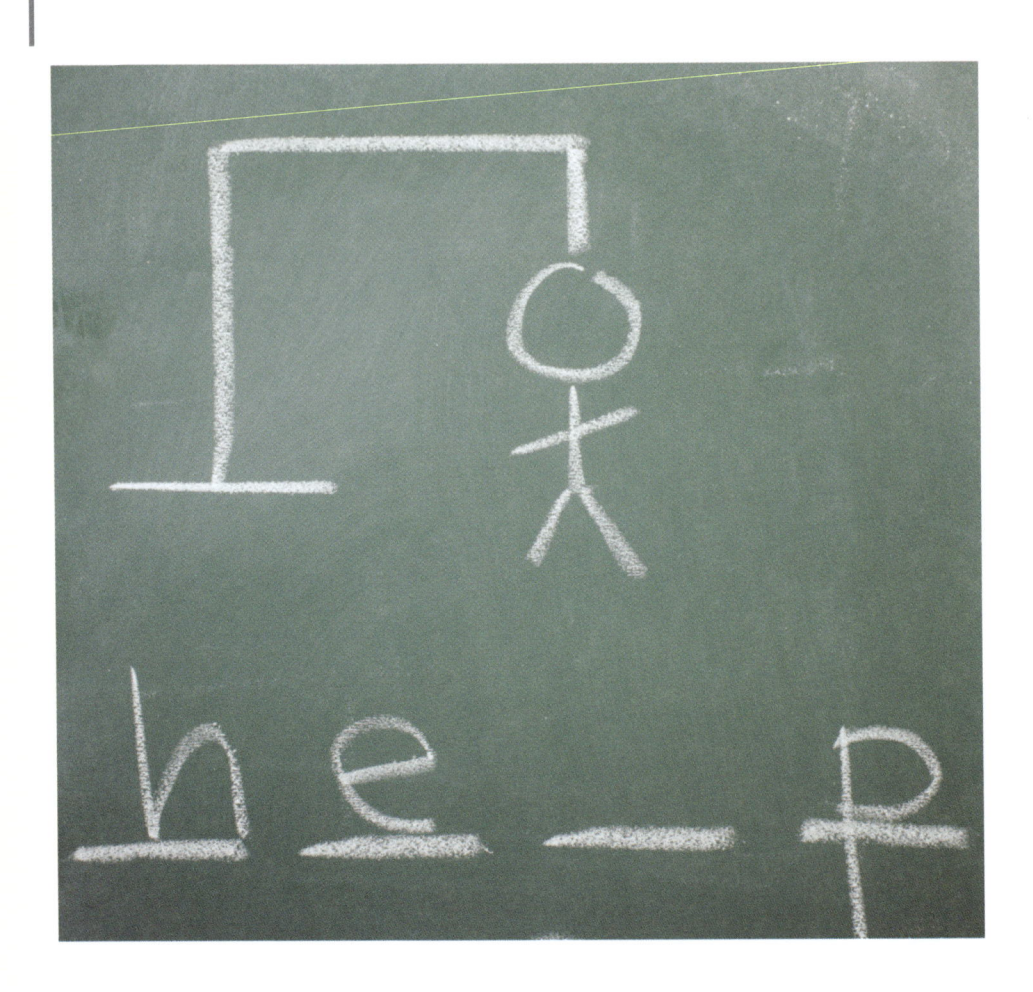

Opening (10 minutes)

❏ All members individually welcomed to the group by name
❏ Draw attention to the name of the group (on the whiteboard)
❏ Remind everyone of the activity in the last session. As a group, sing together the group's 'theme song', led by song leader (use song book or CD)
❏ Discuss day, month, year, season, weather, time, name and address of the place you are in (use whiteboard)
❏ Discuss something currently in the news (use a newspaper, magazine or photograph).

Warm up

❏ Play a soft-ball game for a few minutes – when throwing the ball, people may either state their own name, or, for the more able, the name of the person they are throwing the ball to. Ask members to say their favourite board game.

Making a difference **2**

Main activity (25 to 30 minutes)

Your ideas

Suggested activities:
- Word identification game ('hangman'), involving the recognition and use of letters and words:
  - Draw a number of dashes for each letter of a word and ask the group to guess the letters
  - Incorrect letters contribute to the drawing of a 'hangman' and losing the game
  - The group is required to guess the word
  - Give a category clue (e.g. 'type of drink') if needed
- Prepare a large-size crossword or word search (on A3 paper) – with the difficulty level geared to the group's ability
- Word game 'taboo': Ask a member of the group to explain the card word without being able to use the word, the others in the group have to guess the word.

Triggers

- White board
- Large size crosswords
- Taboo game.

Closing (10 to 15 minutes)

❏ Thank everyone individually for attending and contributing to the session
❏ Summarise the discussion and ideas raised – seek feedback
❏ Sing theme song again
❏ Reminder of time and content of next session
❏ Farewells.

SESSION SEVENTEEN | **Food slogans/ads**

Your ideas

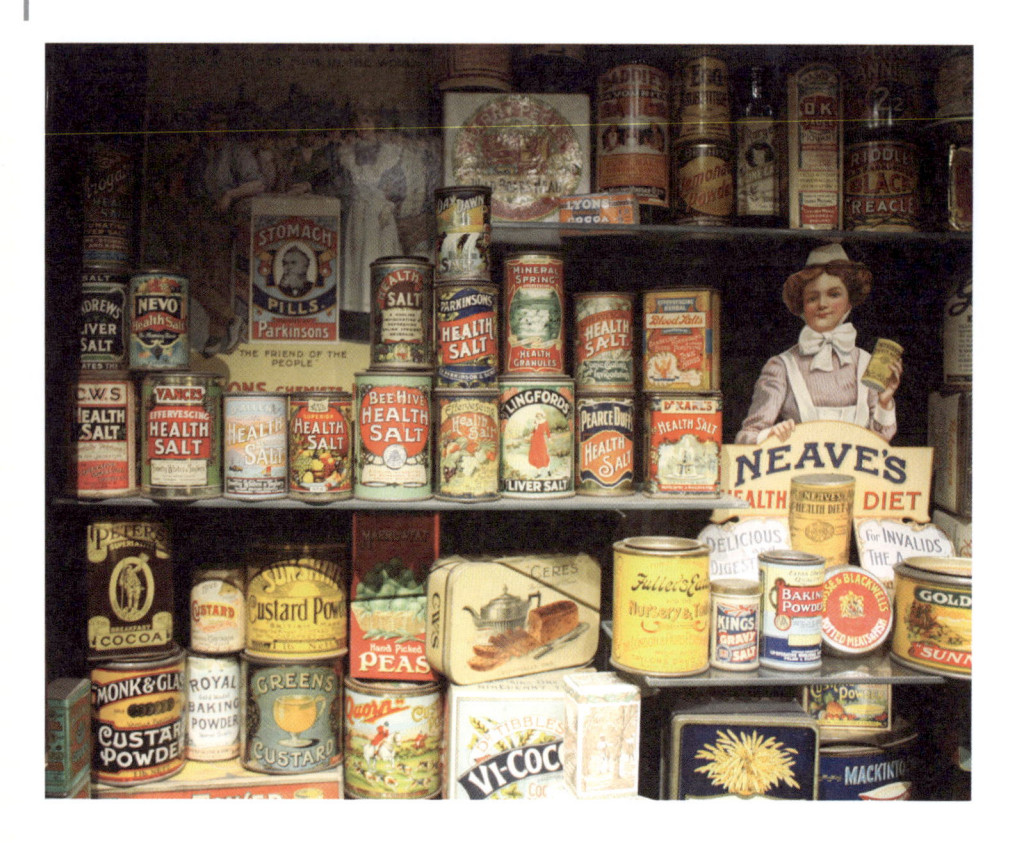

Opening (10 minutes)

❑ All members individually welcomed to the group by name
❑ Draw attention to the name of the group (on the whiteboard)
❑ Remind everyone of the activity in the last session. As a group, sing together the group's 'theme song', led by song leader (use song book or CD)
❑ Discuss day, month, year, season, weather, time, name and address of the place you are in (use whiteboard)
❑ Discuss something currently in the news (use a newspaper, magazine or photograph).

Warm up

❑ Play a soft-ball game for a few minutes – when throwing the ball, people may either state their own name, or, for the more able, the name of the person they are throwing the ball to. As the main activity is going to be 'food', ask members to say their favourite type of food: gastro pub food, Chinese, Italian, Indian, Greek, homemade food etc., or favourite course of a meal: starter, main, dessert.

MAINTENANCE CST SESSIONS

Main activity (25 to 30 minutes)

Your ideas

Suggested activities:
- Brainstorm food categories on the whiteboard, listing as many as possible in each category (e.g. Indian, Chinese, British, Spanish, Italian). Generate discussion about the different ones, which ones are liked and disliked
- Using food advertised from the past compare them with current advertisements. What do they still have in common and what is different? Has the way people feel attracted by a food product changed over the years? Do we look for the same kind of food today?
- Show food advertisements from the past and discuss opinions about them in the group. What do we like or dislike about them? Would we buy that product? You can also ask the group to categorise the advertisements in groups, e.g. vegetables, fruits, conserves, and so on
- Show food advertisement cards and real, or replicas of, food miniatures and ask the group to match them together and categorise them in groups.

Triggers

- Food groceries
- Board
- List of food items
- Food advertisements from Robert Opie collection.

Closing (10 to 15 minutes)

❏ Thank everyone individually for attending and contributing to the session.
❏ Summarise the discussion and ideas raised – seek feedback
❏ Sing theme song again
❏ Reminder of time and content of next session
❏ Farewells.

Making a difference 2

SESSION EIGHTEEN | # Associated words

Your ideas

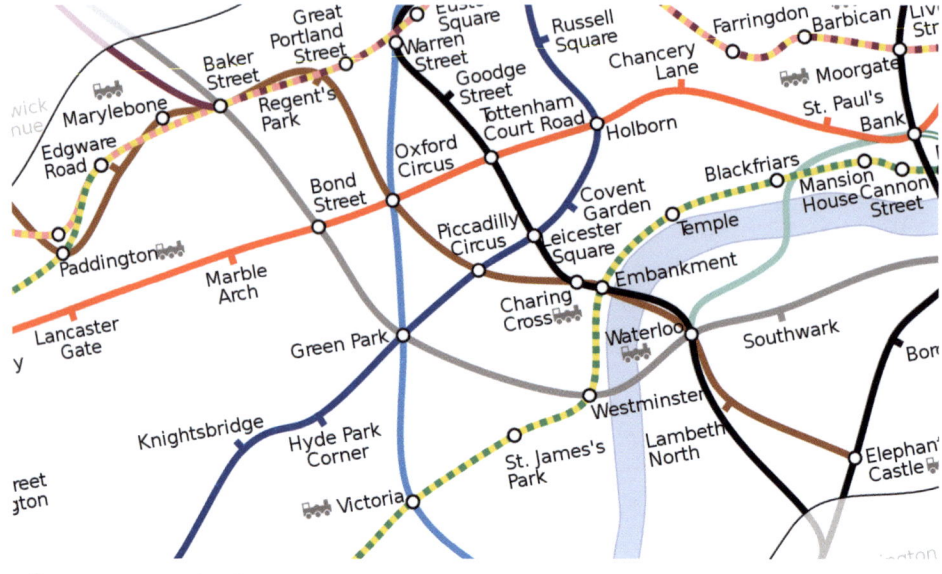

Opening (10 minutes)

- ❏ All members individually welcomed to the group by name
- ❏ Draw attention to the name of the group (on the whiteboard)
- ❏ Remind everyone of the activity in the last session. As a group, sing together the group's 'theme song', led by song leader (use song book or CD)
- ❏ Discuss day, month, year, season, weather, time, name and address of the place you are in (use whiteboard)
- ❏ Discuss something currently in the news (use a newspaper, magazine or photograph).

Warm up

- ❏ Play a soft-ball game for a few minutes – when throwing the ball, people may either state their own name, or, for the more able, the name of the person they are throwing the ball to. Ask members to share with a group a feeling they might be having at the moment.

Main activity (25 to 30 minutes)

Suggested activities:

- Sentence completion task: group members are asked to supply the missing word in a number of phrases. These can include amounts (e.g. a cup of...), famous couples (e.g. Laurel and...), famous places (e.g. Westminster...), proverbs (e.g. 'a stitch in time...'). Discussion can also be generated after the completion of the meaning of some proverbs
- Song completion: present the first few words of a song (e.g.

'we'll meet again….') and ask the group to sing a few lines
- Using maps of the London Underground, London or Britain, ask the group to recall recognised Underground stations, cities or boroughs beginning with a particular letter.

Triggers

- Missing words cards
- Visual maps.

Your ideas

Closing (10 to 15 minutes)

❏ Thank everyone individually for attending and contributing to the session
❏ Summarise the discussion and ideas raised – seek feedback
❏ Sing theme song again
❏ Reminder of time and content of next session
❏ Farewells.

Amounts

Cup of	tea / coffee
Loaf of	bread
Slice of	bread, cake, ham, life etc.
Jug of	water, milk, beer etc.
Pint of	milk, beer etc.
Litre of	petrol
Reel of	cotton
Ball of	wool
Pair of	shoes, trousers, glasses
Bucket of	water, sand

Couples

Laurel and	Hardy
Morecambe and	Wise
Marks and	Spencer
Little and	Large
Crosse and	Blackwell

Places

Westminster	Abbey, Bridge
Buckingham	Palace
Windsor	Castle
Trafalgar	Square
Piccadilly	Circus
Nelson's	Column
Waterloo	Bridge, Station
Canterbury	Cathedral
Charing	Cross
New	York, Orleans, -castle
Times	Square
Capitol	Hill

Proverbs

A stitch in time	saves nine
Make hay while	the sun shines
A watched kettle never	boils
The grass is always greener	on the other side
A bird in the hand is worth	two in the bush
Strike while the iron is	hot
Many hands	make light work
Too many cooks	spoil the broth
Don't put all your eggs	in one basket
Absence makes the heart	grow fonder
Out of sight	out of mind
Don't cry over	spilt milk
Don't cut off your nose	to spite your face
Don't have too many irons	in the fire
Don't look a gift horse	in the mouth
Be careful what you wish for,	you might just get it
Beauty is	in the eye of the beholder
Beauty is	only skin deep
Beggars can't be	choosers
Better late than	never
Better safe than	sorry
A friend in need	is a friend indeed
After a storm	comes a calm
After dinner sit a while	after supper walk a mile
A good beginning makes	a good ending
Charity begins	at home
History repeats	itself
Home is	where the heart is
Home is	where you hang your hat
Honesty is	the best policy
Honey catches more flies	than vinegar

SESSION NINETEEN | **Orientation**

Your ideas

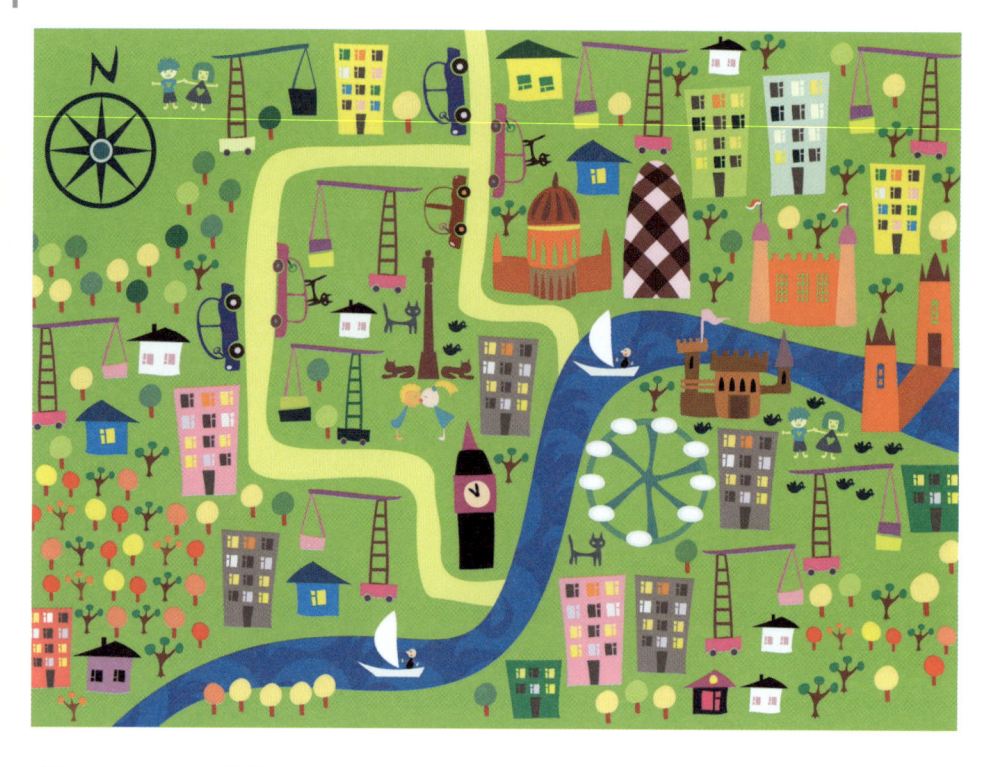

Opening (10 minutes)

- All members individually welcomed to the group by name
- Draw attention to the name of the group (on the whiteboard)
- Remind everyone of the activity in the last session. As a group, sing together the group's 'theme song', led by song leader (use song book or CD)
- Discuss day, month, year, season, weather, time, name and address of the place you are in (use whiteboard)
- Discuss something currently in the news (use a newspaper, magazine or photograph).

Warm up

- Play a soft-ball game for a few minutes – when throwing the ball, people may either state their own name, or, for the more able, the name of the person they are throwing the ball to. As the main activity is going to be 'orientation', ask members to say their favourite place in the world or country or holiday.

Making a difference **2**

MAINTENANCE CST SESSIONS

Main activity (25 to 30 minutes)

Your ideas

Suggested activities:
- Depending on how 'local' group members are, construct a map of the UK, local area or make a floorplan of the care home on whiteboard. Fill in the 'maps' by asking the group to suggest different places or landmarks, such as a favourite seaside destination on the UK map, or the post office in a local area map, or the dining room on the floor plan of the home, and draw them in the appropriate position. Some towns and cities have 'then and now' photograph books, documenting changes during the 20th century – use one of these to stimulate discussion if most members know the area
- Mark on a large map where group members were born and discuss whether people have moved from area to area. If members have travelled abroad, use a map of the world to identify different places. Discuss how long journeys take, how far apart places are and what their transport links and landmarks are.

Triggers

- A3 laminated maps
- Maps you can draw on
- Cavallini & Co Bon Voyage assorted postcards; www.cavallini.com/postcards.html.

Closing (10 to 15 minutes)

❏ Thank everyone individually for attending and contributing to the session
❏ Summarise the discussion and ideas raised – seek feedback
❏ Sing theme song again
❏ Reminder of time and content of next session
❏ Farewell.

SESSION TWENTY

Using money (video clips)

Your ideas

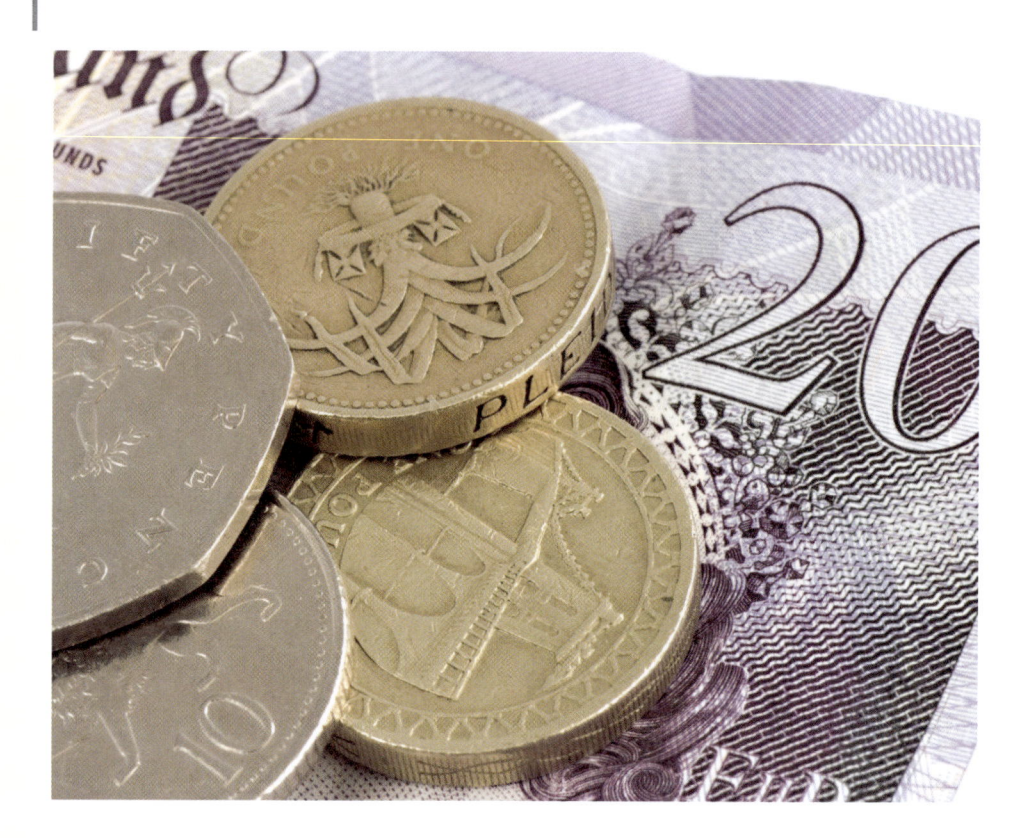

Opening (10 minutes)

❏ All members individually welcomed to the group by name
❏ Draw attention to the name of the group (on the whiteboard)
❏ Remind everyone of the activity in the last session. As a group, sing together the group's 'theme song', led by song leader (use song book or CD)
❏ Discuss day, month, year, season, weather, time, name and address of the place you are in (use whiteboard)
❏ Discuss something currently in the news (use a newspaper, magazine or photograph).

Warm up

❏ Play a soft-ball game for a few minutes – when throwing the ball, people may either state their own name, or, for the more able, the name of the person they are throwing the ball to. Ask members to say whether they would prefer notes to coins, or old money to new money, or would prefer to have euros or pounds in the UK, and the reasons behind their answers.

MAINTENANCE CST SESSIONS

Main activity (25 to 30 minutes)

Your ideas

Suggested activities:
- Use laminated cut-outs of common objects from a catalogue (or actual objects), with prices on the back. Tasks could involve guessing the prices, adding up the prices (how much will the total bill be?), or matching the price tag with the object
- Old and new coins: have examples of each and compare them.
- Changes in prices/values: how much did people get paid for what they did? How much was their first pay packet? What can you get today for £5? How much did a loaf of bread cost when they were young and now?
- Select a commercial advert (can be from a magazine or TV) which shows the sale price of a product. Discuss which option they would take, the 'buy one get one free' or the 50% off offer. Stimulate discussion by asking opinions about the advert. What do they think is going to sell, what do they think about the product, would they buy it?
- Collect different 'house for sale' brochures from local estate agents or off the internet (www.findaproperty.co.uk). Print multiple copies so that each participant can have their own copy. Discuss within the group opinions about the house, number of bedrooms, quality of the house and location. Ask a member to make an offer for the house and the other members can say whether they would make a higher or lower offer. Show the asking price of the house to participants and encourage a conversation about their opinions on the asking price for the house.

Triggers
- Old and new coins
- TV/magazine advertisements
- Laminated cut-outs of common objects from a catalogue
- 'House for sale' brochure.

Closing (10 to 15 minutes)

❏ Thank everyone individually for attending and contributing to the session
❏ Summarise the discussion and ideas raised – seek feedback
❏ Sing theme song again
❏ Reminder of time and content of next session
❏ Farewells.

SESSION TWENTY-ONE

Word game

Your ideas

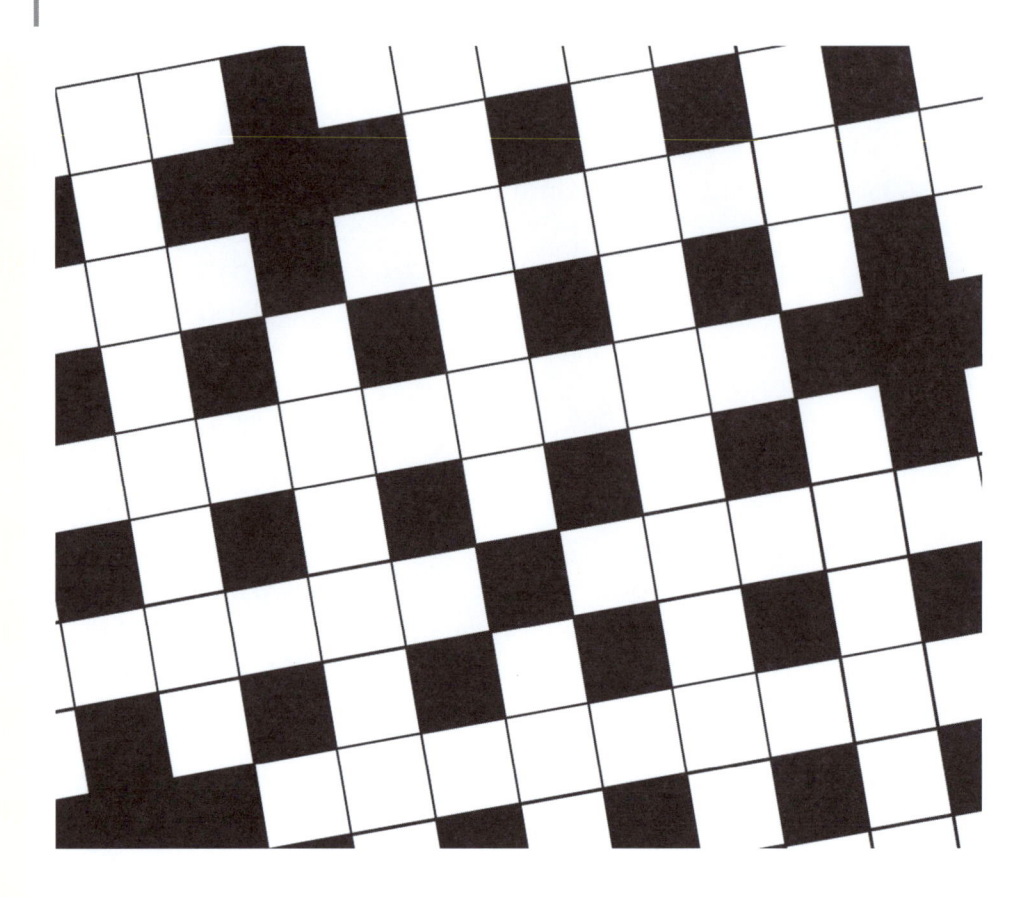

Please refer to session 16 on page 48 to remind yourself of the structure and examples given for this session.

SESSION TWENTY-TWO | **Household treasures**

Your ideas

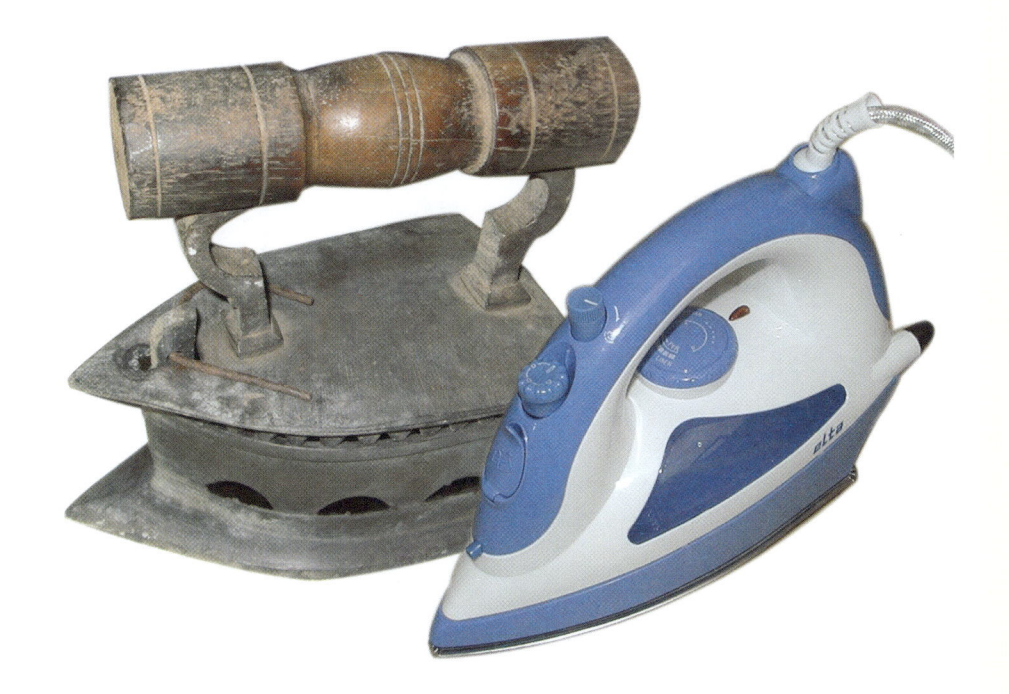

Please refer to session 10 on page 36 to remind yourself of the structure and examples given for this session.

Making a difference 2

SESSION TWENTY-THREE | # My life (occupations)

Your ideas

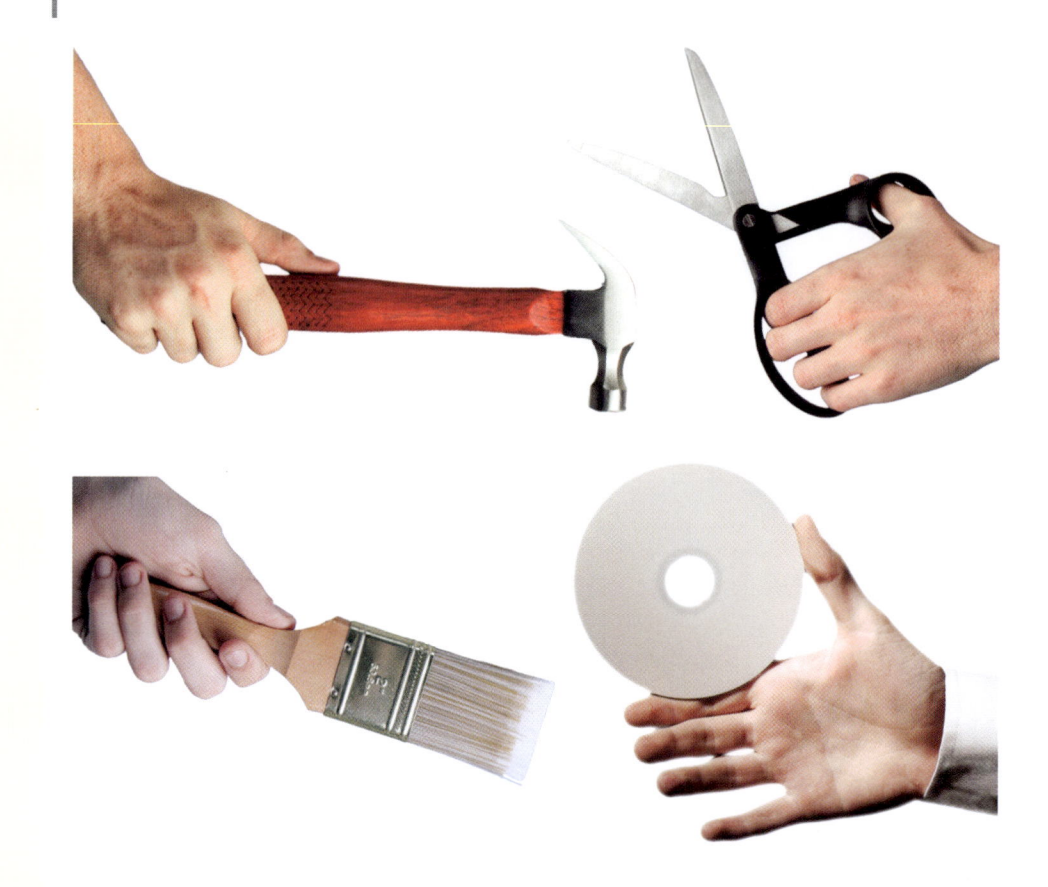

Opening (10 minutes)

❏ All members individually welcomed to the group by name
❏ Draw attention to the name of the group (on the whiteboard)
❏ Remind everyone of the activity in the last session. As a group, sing together the group's 'theme song', led by song leader (use song book or CD)
❏ Discuss day, month, year, season, weather, time, name and address of the place you are in (use whiteboard)
❏ Discuss something currently in the news (use a newspaper, magazine or photograph).

Warm up

❏ Play a soft-ball game for a few minutes – when throwing the ball, people may either state their own name, or, for the more able, the name of the person they are throwing the ball to. As the main activity is going to be 'my life and occupations', ask members to say a job they have had.

MAINTENANCE CST SESSIONS

Main activity (25 to 30 minutes)

Your ideas

Suggested activities:
- From a selection of drawings of occupations ask members to choose the one that it is closest to their occupation or profession
- Ask members to make a list of objects that would describe the work or profession they had
- Present a list of objects and ask participants to describe occupations that come to mind when looking at the objects
- Members can describe their profession and other members in the group can try to guess it
- Organise a selection of pictures of occupations according to categories, for example, manual work, academic work, health related work, or perhaps jobs which are male or female oriented.

Triggers

- Cards with different occupations and uniforms
- Objects which bring to mind different occupations.

Closing (10 to 15 minutes)

❏ Thank everyone individually for attending and contributing to the session
❏ Summarise the discussion and ideas raised – seek feedback
❏ Sing theme song again
❏ Reminder of time and content of next session
❏ Farewells.

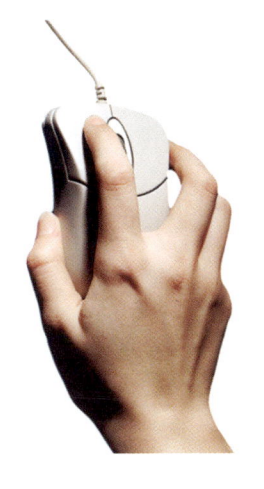

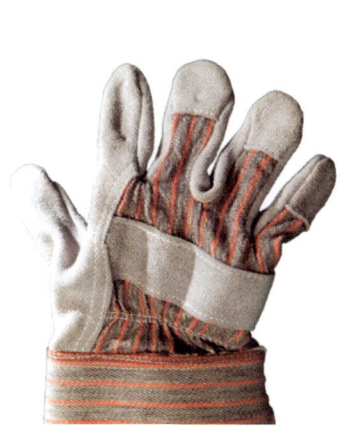

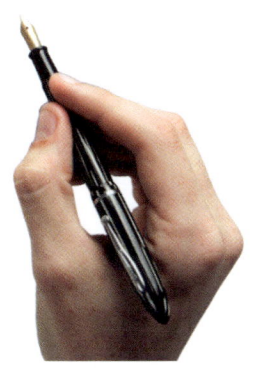

Making a difference 2

SESSION TWENTY-FOUR | # Useful tips (healthy living)

Your ideas

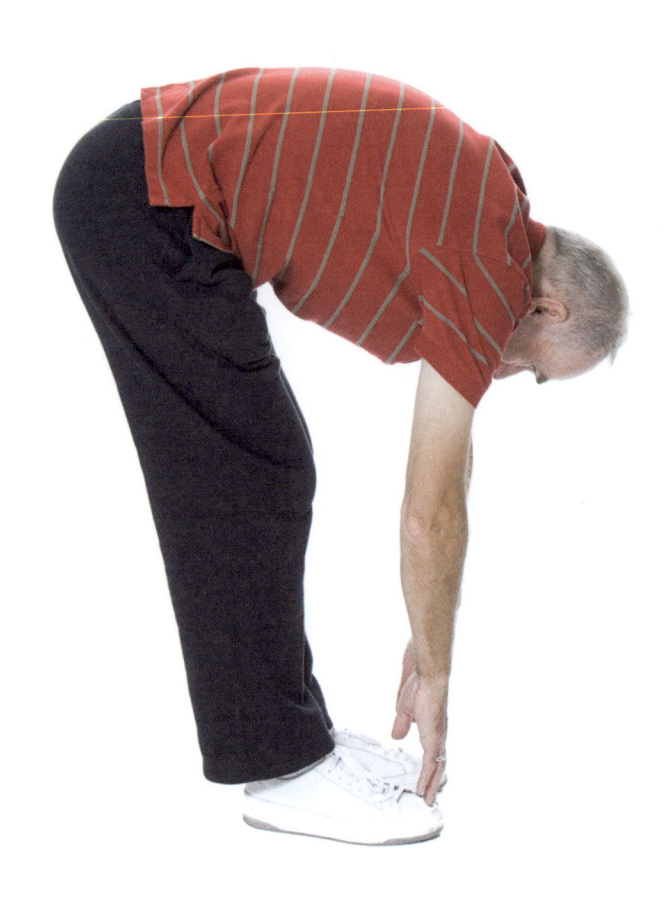

Opening (10 minutes)

- All members individually welcomed to the group by name
- Draw attention to the name of the group (on the whiteboard)
- Remind everyone of the activity in the last session. As a group, sing together the group's 'theme song', led by song leader (use song book or CD)
- Discuss day, month, year, season, weather, time, name and address of the place you are in (use whiteboard)
- Discuss something currently in the news (use a newspaper, magazine or photograph).

Warm up

- Play a soft-ball game for a few minutes – when throwing the ball, people may either state their own name, or, for the more able, the name of the person they are throwing the ball to. As the main activity is going to be 'useful advice and tips about healthy living' ask participants about the area of health they believe is most important, about diet, exercise and lifestyle. Use prompt cards as needed.

References and further reading

Aguirre E, Spector A, Orrell M (2009) Cognitive Stimulation Therapy (CST): Past and future of an evidence based therapy. *Signpost Journal of Dementia and Mental Health Care of Older People* 13 1.

Aguirre E, Spector A, Hoe J, Russell T I, Knapp M, Woods RT, Orrell M (2010) Maintenance Cognitive Stimulation Therapy (CST) for dementia: A single-blind, multi-centre, randomized controlled trial of Maintenance CST vs. CST for dementia. *Trials* 11 46.

Aguirre E, Spector A, Hoe J, Streater A, Russell IT, Woods RT, Orrell M (2011) Development of an evidence-based extended programme of maintenance cognitive stimulation therapy (CST) for people with dementia. *Non-pharmacological Therapies in Dementia Journal* 1 (1) 61-70.

Aguirre E, Spector A, Streater A, Burnell K, Orrell M (2011) "Service users' involvement in the development of a maintenance Cognitive Stimulation Therapy (CST) programme: A comparison of the views of people with dementia, staff and family carers". *Dementia Journal* 4 10.

Breuil V, De Rotrou J, Forette F, Tortrat D, Ganansia Ganem A, Frambourt A, Moulin F, Boller F (1994) Cognitive Stimulation of patients with dementia: Preliminary results. *International Journal of Geriatric Psychiatry* 9 (3) 211-217.

Clare L, Moniz-Cook E, Orrell M, Spector A, Woods B (2004) Cognitive rehabilitation and cognitive training for early-stage Alzheimer's disease and vascular dementia. In: *The Cochrane Library*. Chichester: Wiley.

Knapp M, Thorgrimsen L, Patel A, Spector A, Hallam A, Woods B, Orrell M (2006) Cognitive Stimulation Therapy for people with dementia: Cost Effectiveness Analysis. *British Journal of Psychiatry* 188 574-580.

Medical Research Council (2008) *A framework for development and evaluation of RCTs for complex interventions to improve health.* London.

National Institute of Clinical Excellence (2006) Clinical Guideline 42. In: *Supporting people with dementia and their carers in health and social care.* London: Department of Health.

Orrell M, Spector A, Thorgrimsen L, Woods B (2005) A pilot study examining the effectiveness of maintenance Cognitive Stimulation Therapy (MCST) for people with dementia. *International Journal of Geriatric Psychiatry* 20 446-451.

Small GW (2002) What we need to know about age related memory loss. *British Medical Journal* 324 1502-1505.

Spector A, Davies S, Woods B, Orrell M (1998) Reality orientation for dementia: a review of the evidence for its effectiveness. In: *The Cochrane Library 4* Oxford Update Software.

Spector A, Gardner C, Orrell M (2011) The impact of Cognitive Stimulation Therapy groups on people with dementia: views from participants, their carers and group facilitators. *Aging & Mental Health*, 15, July 4.

Spector A, Orrell M, Davies S, Woods B (2001) Can reality orientation be rehabilitated? Development and piloting of an evidence based programme of cognition-based therapies for people with dementia. *Neuropsychological Rehabilitation* 11 (3-4) 377-397.

Spector A, Thorgrimsen L, Woods B, Royan L, Davies S, Butterworth M, Orrell M (2003) Efficacy of an evidence-based cognitive stimulation therapy programme for people with dementia: Randomised Controlled Trial. *British Journal of Psychiatry* 183 248-254.

Spector A, Aguirre E, Orrell M (2010) Translating Research Into Practice: A Pilot Study Examining the Use of Cognitive Stimulation Therapy (CST) after a one-day training course. *Non-pharmacological Therapies in Dementia Journal* 1 (1) 61-70.

Woods RT (2002) Non-pharmacological techniques. In: Qizilbash N. *Evidence-based dementia practice.* Oxford: Blackwell 428-446.

Woods B, Aguirre E, Orrell M, Spector A (2011) Cognitive Stimulation Therapy programme for dementia. Database of Systematic Reviews (in press).

MAINTENANCE CST SESSIONS

Main activity (25 to 30 minutes)

Your ideas

Suggested activities:
- Using a book about healthy customs and remedies from the past or a book about current healthy living hints and tips encourage discussion and ask participants about how to:
  – Eat a healthy diet
  – Keep exercising regularly, with examples
  – Keep a healthy lifestyle
  – Sleep well
  – Develop memory strategies.
- Ask participants about differences in perceptions about healthy living between the past and now. What used to be acceptable and now is not? In their opinion, what do they think is the healthiest way of living? What do they think about healthy living tips recommended in the past and now? What are the differences and similarities?
- As this is the final session, the group can create their own healthy tips book to take home with them after this final session.

Triggers

- Household Hints & Tips by Linda Gray: www.amazon.co.uk
- Traditional Remedies by Linda Gray: www.amazon.co.uk
- Grandma's Household Hints And Tips: www.homemade-dessert-recipes.com/helpful-household-hints.html

Closing (10 to 15 minutes)

❏ Thank everyone individually for attending and contributing to the session
❏ Summarise the discussion and ideas raised – seek feedback
❏ Sing theme song for the final time
❏ Farewells.

Making a difference 2